Breastfeeding
A Guide for Midwives

Dora Henschel, RN, RM, MTD, IBCLC
with Sally Inch, RN, RM

Books for Midwives Press
Books for Midwives Press is a joint collaboration
between the Royal College of Midwives and
Haigh and Hochland Publications Ltd

Published by Books for Midwives Press, 174a Ashley Road, Hale, Cheshire, WA15 9SF,
England

© 1996, Dora Henshel with Sally Inch
First edition

ISBN1-898507-12-0

British Library Cataloguing in Publication Data
A catalogue record for this book is available from the British Library

Printed in Great Britain

Contents

Acknowledgements

I want to thank all the investigators whose research I have quoted and whose ideas have contributed to this book.

My interest in breastfeeding can be traced back to my midwifery training, and midwifery tutor, Eileen Snelling, who inspired my interest in postnatal care and breastfeeding in particular. I owe her a great deal of gratitude.

I was fortunate in working with a very experienced midwife for the first ten years after qualifying, the late Olive Rogers. She was a pioneer in the management of breastfeeding. Much of what she taught me has been confirmed by research since then and my gratitude to her will never cease.

I would like to thank the many mothers, colleagues, students and friends from whom I have learned over the years in a variety of ways and for sharing their expertise. In particular, I would like to thank Dr Harold Gamsu, Chloe Fisher, Lea Jamieson, Moyra Heggie, Sandra Lang, Gabrielle Palmer, Sue Saunders, Dr Felicity Savage-King and Dr Mike Woolridge.

Specific thanks are due to Hilary English and Sally Inch for providing the photographs.

My special thanks go to my long-time friend and colleague, Janette Smith, for her constant support and especially for reading and commenting thoughtfully on the early manuscript.

Finally I want to express my profound gratitude to Sally Inch who became involved with this book towards the end of its gestation. I greatly appreciate her professional knowledge and the efficient way in which she has worked on this book.

Introduction

The time will come when diligent research over long periods will bring to light things which now lie hidden ... when our when our descendants will be amazed that we did not know things that are plain to them...
Seneca, Natural Questions, Book 7, first century.

This book is concerned with the advantages of breastmilk and breastfeeding in the first few weeks of life of the normal healthy baby. It also includes information about national and international initiatives which project, promote and support breastfeeding.

Any book that challenges entrenched methods of practice may arouse some resentment. The object of this book is to give the current supporting evidence of the need to question and change some professionals most closely associated with this aspect of childbearing. It takes knowledge and confidence to give adequate support to empower women to breastfeed.

During the last decade breastmilk, lactation and breastfeeding have caught the attention of researchers as their importance for the infant is beginning to be understood, not only from a practical, but from a biological and scientific point of view (Over 1, 000 papers were published on these subjects in 1993).

Breastfeeding is also, and always will be, a very emotional subject. Prejudices, opinions and controversy still abound, but the need for more education as an important step forward is being recognized and addressed.

A number of post-certificate courses have been developed. These have been arranged through the Department of Health, WHO/UNICEF, Departments of Midwifery Studies as well as individuals.

It is hoped that in the near future all statutory courses will include breastfeeding as in-depth subject to ensure that all health professionals are well-informed, and that this book will be considered a useful resource.

CHAPTER ONE

Breastmilk – A Species-Specific Food

Setting the scene

Mammals have populated the earth for some 60 million years (Carrington, 1963). They have been through various stages of evolution. Some early species became extinct and today some 3500 different mammals are in existence. Their early survival depends on the species-specific milk the mother provides. In the last 100,000 years or so, humans have become the supreme mammals and their young also need the species-specific milk of their mother.

The body of the human mother prepares for lactation early in pregnancy. With the proliferation of glandular tissue, the breasts grow in size. The accompanying tenderness, tingling and heaviness are often the first sign that conception has taken place. Thus nature prepares very early for the provision of nourishment of the newborn infant and it seems illogical that this special fluid should be so frequently ignored for another mammal's milk.

The vast amount of scientific data which exists about the 'unique significance' of human milk and breastfeeding (Jelliffe and Jelliffe, 1988) confirms a 'gut feeling' in the population that 'breast feeding is best feeding' (Graffy, 1992). Yet in spite of this not all health professionals feel that breastfeeding should be promoted. For example, when Bruce (1991) asked midwives whether a feeding policy should promote and encourage breastfeeding, he found they responded as follows:

* 27 per cent supported a breastfeeding promotion policy

* 61 per cent felt the policy should be neutral

* 12 per cent said there should be no policy.

The main reason for not promoting breastfeeding was the fear that guilt might be induced among mothers who were unable or unwilling to breastfeed. This response may have been due to:

* lack of knowledge about breastmilk and how it differs from formula

- lack of knowledge about the growing body of evidence of the disadvantages to the infant of being fed a breastmilk substitute

- their own feelings of inadequacy when called upon to give practical help with breastfeeding (Palmer, 1993).

Scientific data on human milk

Human milk has been called 'the Gold Standard' for the nourishment of human babies, as it provides all the essential ingredients needed for health and growth. It differs considerably from the milks of other mammals (see Table 1). By the end of the last century the relationship between the nutrient content and the growth rate of difference species had already been noted. For example, it takes (on average) 180 days for the human baby to double it's birthweight, whereas the calf achieves this in 47 and a goat in 19 days (Hambreus, 1977).

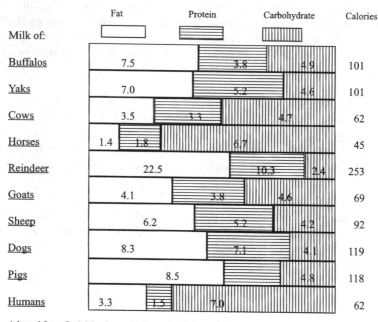

Adapted from fig.1.1 In: *Breastfeeding - the Biological Option*. Ebrahim GJ. 1979.
Educational low priced book scheme with MacMillan.

Table 1. Composition of various milks (per 100mls)

Breastmilk is a complex fluid, with more than 200 known constituents (Blanc, 1981). Greatly improved laboratory facilities and techniques and the availability of electron-microscopes have taken scientists into the 'micro-world' of human milk. As analytical techniques have improved with these facilities, the knowledge of its biochemistry has become vast (Lawrence, 1989). In their introduction to *Programmes to Promote Breastfeeding*, Derrick and Patrice Jelliffe (1988) stated that 'the biochemical differences in human milk, cows' milk and infant formula have been absurdly simplified in paediatric and other text books'.

They continued: 'In fact the only real similarities between the three are that they are whitish in colour and contain water and lactose'.

	Carbohydrate %	Fat %	Protein %	Energy kcal
Human milk	7.0	3.8	0.9	70
Cow's milk	4.8	3.7	3.7	68

Table 2. Comparison of mature human milk with cows' milk
(Adapted from Hambraeus, L. (1977). *Paediatric Clin North Am*; 24: p.17.)

(The differences between this table and the table opposite are probably due to differences in the timing of milk collection (fat) and the inclusion of non-nutritive proteins.)

The uniqueness of breastmilk

Breastmilk is a living, cellular fluid, constantly changing to meet the needs of the infant. It changes from:

• colostrum to transitional then mature milk

• the beginning to the end of a feed

• morning to evening.

Although it varies from mother to mother, depending to some extent on her nutritional state and the foods she eats (National Academy of Sciences, 1991), the milk of the

Days postpartum	1	2	4	14	28
Ingredient:					
Yield (g/24h)	50	190	625	110	1250
Lactose (g/dl)	2	2.5	3.2	3.3	3.5
Fat (g/dl)	1.2	1.5	2.5	2.3	2.9
Protein (g/dl)	3.2	1.7	1.1	0.8	0.9

Table 3. Amount and composition of human colostrum and milk from day 1-28

average, well nourished mother will contain the following:-
(Adapted from Saint, L., Smith, M., Hartmann, P.E. (1984). *British Journal of Nutrition*

52: p.87.)

Breastmilk also varies from one woman to another in relation to the protective factors it contains, which in turn will depend on the infectious diseases to which a woman has been exposed.

For example, if the mother has been exposed to cholera, her milk contains antibodies against this disease (Glass, 1983). The highest concentration of these protective factors occurs in the first few days of lactation (Goldman, 1989).

Amazingly enough, a mother's body responds to the premature birth of her baby by increasing the secretion of protective factors in her milk still further (Jain, 1991).

Composition of human milk

The ratio of total solids to fluid is 12:88. The well-fed baby receives not only all the nourishment but also all the fluid it needs - from its mother's milk.

Colostrum

Due to a ten-fold higher carotene content than mature milk, colostrum is yellow in colour (Lawrence, 1989).

It differs from mature milk in that it contains:

* more protein, including a high concentration of IgA

* a higher concentration of fat-soluble vitamins A and E

* less fat and lactose

* a higher concentration of leucocytes than are present in mature milk (Buescher, 1986).

Mature milk

Carbohydrate

Lactose, a sugar found only in milk, is the main carbohydrate constituent in human milk (Acre, 1989) and provides 37 per cent of the energy provided by breastmilk (Department of Health, 1994). It is a disaccharide which splits on digestion into two monosaccharides, glucose and galactose, the latter being essential for central nervous system development.

As well as aiding calcium and iron absorption, lactose also promotes intestinal colonization with the Lacto-bacillus bifidus, whose growth is further encouraged by a nitrogen containing oligosaccharide, the bifidus factor. This organism has the ability to break down lactose into lactic acid and acetic acid (Worthington-Roberts, 1993). The acid medium created in the gut by the lactobacillus is another factor which inhibits the growth of enteropathogenic organisms.

Fats

Fat is the most variable constituent in human milk and provides 50 per cent of the energy of breastmilk. The fat concentration rises as the feed proceeds, with the hind milk four to five times richer than the foremilk (Acre, 1989). The main constituents (98 per cent) of the fat are triglycerides. Other forms of fat are small amounts of phospholipids, cholesterol, glycolipids and free fatty acids. The fatty acid composition is influenced by the woman's diet (Harzer, 1984). The general change from animal fats to more plant and seed fats/oils in the diet has increased these polyunsaturated fats in human milk (Lawrence, 1994). Two of these compounds, linoleic and linolenic acid, are converted into longer-chain polyunsaturated fatty acids, notably arachadonic acid and docosahexanoic acid. These are required for prostaglandin synthesis (Lawrence, 1994b) and are essential for the development of the nervous system and the quality of the myelin laid down (Dick, 1976).

This century a new type of fat has been developed containing trans fatty acids. Trans fatty acids are not present in nature but are formed by the process of hydrogenation which saturates or harden oils so that they become solid at room temperature. This makes them more suitable for food processing. Trans-fatty acids are stored in body fat and have been found in human milk at levels of up to 18 per cent of the total fatty acid concentration (Chappell, 1985).

There is still considerable controversy about the biological effects of trans fatty acids (Lawrence, 1994c). They adversely affect lipid metabolism and this has the potential to cause detrimental health effects (Sinclair, 1992). It is possible that they may impair the synthesis of prostaglandins, which regulate many biological functions, by blocking the conversion of essential fatty acids. However, whether their presence in human milk affects the health of the child is not yet known.

Protein nitrogens

Protein is required for growth of the baby. If energy intake is low, it is also used to provide energy. Mature milk has the lowest protein concentration amongst mammals (Akre, 1990). In human milk, the amount of whey protein, which forms a soft, flocculent and easily digested curd in the infant's stomach, is four times greater than that of casein, which forms a harder curd (Hambraeus, 1976). A large portion of the whey protein consists of *anti-infective factors*, the components of which are:

> 'lactalbumin, immunoglobulins, lactoferrin, lysozyme, enzymes, hormones and growth factors' (Lawson, 1992).

Lactoferrin is the major whey protein fraction and binds iron, making it unavailable to iron dependent bacteria i.e. Escherichia Coli. It has been suggested that additional iron in the diet of a breastfed baby may interfere with this bacteriostatic function.

Lactoferrin is valued so highly that genetic engineering research is attempting to transfer the human gene responsible for the production of lactoferrin into freshly fertilized bovine ova to activate its production by the cow's milk producing tissues.

Secretory IgA is the principal immunoglobulin. It functions as a valuable defence mechanism in the gut by preventing the entry of viruses and bacteria into the mucosa of the intestinal wall (Lawrence, 1994d).

Epidermal Growth Factor, (EGF) a polypeptide, was identified in 1963 by Professor Stanley Cohen, for which he subsequently received the Nobel Prize. It stimulates the proliferation of epidermal and epithelial tissues and stimulates cell proliferation of the lining of the gut. EGF can now be produced synthetically at great expense and has been used in clinical trials to treat severe burn injuries. It is freely available to the baby, in breastmilk!

Lysozyme, together with other components in human milk, breaks down and kills susceptible bacteria (Butte, 1984). During the first six months of lactation, the concentration of lysozyme gradually increases (Prenticem, 1984).

Non-protein nitrogens

Three of these important compounds are *Taurine, Nucleotides and Carnitine*

Taurine, a free amino acid, virtually absent from cows' milk, is important for bile acid conjugation, brain and retinal development.

Nucleotides are essential precursors for DNA and RNA, and are important for the function of cell membranes and the normal development of the brain. Nucleotides have also been suggested as co-factors for the growth of bifido bacteria, which reduce the presence of pathogens, such as Escherichia coli, in the faecal flora (Balmer, 1994).

Carnitine is essential for the catabolism of long-chain fatty acids. It enables fatty acids and ketone bodies to be oxidized to provide alternative fuels to glucose. This important function has relevance to neonatal hypoglycaemia and is currently being investigated (Hawdon, 1993).

The major minerals and trace elements are:

* sodium
* calcium
* phosphorus
* magnesium
* zinc
* copper
* iron.

The quantities and ratios of all these substances are species-specific and the mineral content of human milk and cow's milk differ considerably. In 1976, strict controls for the production of breastmilk substitutes were introduced by the Department of Health and the Ministry of Agriculture, Fisheries and Food (MAFF, 1981).

This was in response to the discovery that excess sodium and phosphorus in the dried milks used for artificially feeding infants were responsible for two serious conditions; hypernatraemia (caused by the excess sodium) and neonatal tetany, due to the high phosphorus content which depressed calcium up-take.

Currently the composition of breastmilk substitutes are controlled by legislation. The European Economic Community Directive 89/398/EEC was replaced in June 1995 by the Infant Formula and Follow-on Formula Regulations (Statutory Instruments 1995 No.7) which detail the range of the amount of each constituent and the permitted sources, for all breastmilk substitutes.

Although the amount of iron is low in human milk, its absorption is highly efficient and iron deficiency in the breastfed infant is rarely observed (Fransson, 1980). Up to 70 per cent of breastmilk iron is absorbed, compared with only ten per cent of the iron in breastmilk substitutes (Saarinnen, 1979). To compensate for this, large amounts of supplemental iron have to be added to the substitutes, which in turn favours the development of pathogenic gut bacteria. Additional iron can also reduce the absorption of two other trace elements, zinc and copper (Oski, 1985).

Vitamins

The supply of vitamins in the breastmilk of a well nourished mother will normally satisfy the infant's requirements for vitamins, with the possible exception of vitamin K (Present day Practice, 1974; Bates, 1985).

VITAMIN A

In industrialized countries mothers are unlikely to lack this vitamin in their diet and consequently in their breastmilk. Vitamin A rich foods, leafy vegetables and yellow and orange fruits and vegetables, are freely available.

Children in less developed countries often suffer from a deficiency in vitamin A, resulting in severe visual impairment and blindness from corneal scarring (Xerophthalmia) (Rahi, 1995).

Morbidity and mortality from measles and diarrhoea is also increased (Ghana VAST Study Team, 1993) when this vitamin is lacking. Projects in various underdeveloped countries have improved this situation by giving mothers high dose vitamin A capsules within four weeks of birth (so that there is no danger of the mother being pregnant and thus no danger of teratogenic effect) to increase her breastmilk retinol concentration for at least eight months (Filteau, 1995).

VITAMIN K

Newborn babies have a low plasma concentration of vitamin K and the baby's gut is sterile at birth, taking several days for the intestinal flora to begin to produce this vitamin. Current research seems to support the proposal that infants are at risk from haemorrhagic disease, if supplemental vitamin K is not given (Croucher, 1994). The risk concerns mainly breastfed babies, as only small quantities of vitamin K are present in breastmilk.

It seems strange that nature may not have provided this vitamin in the necessary quantities to prevent this condition. The explanation for this apparent omission may be that the hindmilk, which contains the vitamin K, is not being obtained by the infant (Kries, 1987). This may be due to poor positioning and/or a restriction in the duration of feeds.

The concentration of vitamin K is higher in colostrum than milk. In a small study, (10 mothers with term infants) the quantity of vitamin K in colostrum and mature milk was measured on days 1, 3, 5, 8, 15, 22, 29 and 36. The concentration of Vitamin K in colostrum (days one-five) was significantly higher (p < 0.001) than that found in mature milk (days 8-36). Considerable variations were found in the quantities between the individual mothers.

The authors emphasized the great importance of an adequate intake of colostrum in the first days of life and stressed that a low intake of colostrum during this time exposed newborn infants to an increased risk of vitamin K deficiency (Kries, 1987), resulting in classic haemorrhagic disease (two to seven days after birth).

The other form, late haemorrhagic disease (one to three months after birth) in exclusively breastfed infants, has been described as a relatively new disease, and an important cause of morbidity and mortality since 1975 (Lane, 1985).

In a discussion paper, Koppe (1989) related the possible cause of this problem to the presence of polychlorobiphenyls (PCBs), polychlorinated dibenzo-p-dioxins (PCDDs) and polychlorinated dibenzofurans (PCDFs) in the breastmilk of mothers, living in industrialized countries. He considered it to be plausible that these substances may interfere with the metabolism in the liver leading to vitamin K deficiency.

Since the 1960s and 1970s 1mg of intramuscular vitamin K (TM: Konakion) has been the standard prophylaxis for babies but it has been a controversial practice since it began (Draper, 1994). The suggestion from the work of Golding (1992) that the use of intramuscular vitamin K is associated with a doubling of the incidence of childhood cancer received much publicity.

The response was to replace intramuscular vitamin K with oral vitamin K, but the wisdom of this has been questioned because of the difficulties of administering a prolonged course of treatment, dose one being at birth, dose two at one to two weeks and dose three at four weeks of age.

Retrospective studies undertaken in Sweden (Ekelund, 1993) and America (American Academy of Pediatrics, 1993) have examined the incidence of childhood cancer in relation to the administration of intramuscular vitamin K and found no increase in malignancy associated with the use of intramuscular vitamin K. Thus the debate on the administration of vitamin K continues.

Enzymes

Breastmilk contains over 20 enzymes, which contribute to digestion and development. Possibly the two most important aids to infant digestion are:

Amylase - which is produced in only very small amounts in the pancreas of the term newborn. It is present in breastmilk throughout lactation and acts on starches, breaking them down into mono and disaccharides.

Lipase - is present only in the milks of humans and gorillas (Akre, 1989). It is activated by bile salts in the duodenum and contributes to the digestion of 30 - 40 per cent of triglycerides. The presence of this enzyme in breastmilk is especially important for the preterm infant, whose pancreatic lipase production is poor.

Conclusion

Such is the importance of human milk to the human infant that in her book, *Breastfeeding - A Guide For The Medical Profession,* Dr. R. Lawrence states categorically:

> 'The clinician should not have to justify the recommendation for breastfeeding, but instead the paediatrician should have to justify the replacement with a cows' milk substitute' (Lawrence, 1994e).

CHAPTER TWO

The Value of Breastmilk for Health

Hardly a month passes without the discovery of a new constituent of breastmilk or some new knowledge about the ratios or concentrations of its components (Goldman, 1987).

On the surface it would appear that the human infant has adapted relatively well to the modified milk of another species. However, as more babies are artificially fed, the problems associated with artificial feeding are becoming more apparent. At the same time, more attention is being given to the methodological design of research studies to make the results more robust (Howie, 1990).

Some of the constituents of breastmilk mentioned in the previous chapter, and which are missing from formulae, are probably responsible for the improved health of the breastfed infants in the studies listed below.

Protection of the infant from infection

Human milk has been called 'a potent immunocompetent agent, containing a rich variety of products, each one of which has a role to play in the immunological protection of the infant' (Ebrahim, 1995). The major agents may overlap and have more than one function.

1.   Antimicrobial factors (e.g. Lysosyme and lactoferrin)
2.   Anti-inflammatory agents (e.g. Lysosyme and lactoferrin)
3.   Other biologically active products (e.g. Oligosaccharides).

The breastfed infant thus receives significantly more protection from disease than his bottlefed counterpart.

Diarrhoea

It is well known that the mortality rate of artificially fed babies in developing countries is high. For example a study from Brazil (Victora et al, 1987) found that:

> 'the relative risk of infant death from common infections was much higher in those who had not been breastfed. After adjusting for confounding variables, those receiving no breastmilk had 14.2 and 3.6 times the risk of death from diarrhoea and respiratory infections, respectively, than those who were breastfed'.

Infant deaths caused by diarrhoea or respiratory infections may be a rare event in an industrialized country but is still a cause for morbidity and misery for both infant and families.

Gastro-intestinal disease was found to be much more prevalent in the artificially fed baby in a study undertaken in Dundee by Howie (1990). Investigating the relationship between infant feeding and infectious illness, he followed the progress of 674 infants, of whom 277 were breastfed for 13 weeks or more. In 130 of these cases, supplements were introduced before 13 weeks and in 97 cases they were not. 27 cases were excluded because of incomplete documentation.

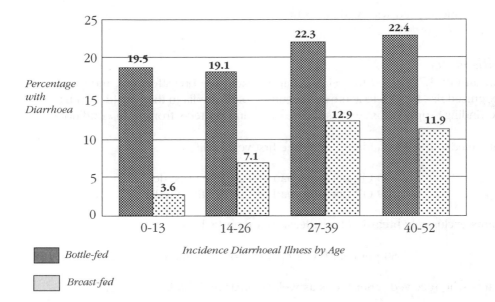

Incidence Diarrhoeal Illness by Age

Bottle-fed

Breast-fed

Prevalence of Infant Diarrhoea up to 1 year by Feeding Pattern 0-13 weeks, Dundee.

The 89 babies who were fully breastfed for 13 weeks or more had substantial protection from gastro-intestinal illness with an incidence of 2.9 per cent (when adjusted for social class, maternal age and parental smoking) compared with the bottle fed and early weaning group whose adjusted rate was 15.7 per cent and 16.7 per cent respectively (A five fold difference).

Gastro-intestinal disease was defined as vomiting or diarrhoea or both, lasting as a discrete illness for 48 hours or more (Chandra, 1979). (Chronic malabsorption was excluded). The study did not assess the degree of illness. It can be assumed, however, that some babies would have to be admitted to hospital for treatment with a considerable cost to the Health Service.

In 1992, in Greater Glasgow, the cost of admitting babies with this condition to hospital was £204,500 for a total of 1382 bed days! (Campbell, 1993).

Respiratory illness

In the same study, Howie (1990) also found smaller, but still statistically significant, reductions in the rates of respiratory disease in babies who were breastfed for as little as 13 weeks.

The adjusted rate for babies:

- fully breastfed for 13 weeks was 25.6 per cent

- partially breastfed for 13 weeks was 24.2 per cent

- artificially fed was 37.0 per cent.

Otitis media

Duncan (1993) assessed the relationship of exclusive breastfeeding, independent of recognized risk factors, to acute and recurrent otitis media in the first 12 months of life. The findings suggest that exclusive breastfeeding protects from both conditions.

Otitis media in 1013 children during the first year of life:

> 476 (47 per cent) had at least one episode
> 169 (17 per cent) had recurrent otitis media

Infants exclusively breastfed for at least four months had:

> 50 per cent fewer episodes of otitis media

Infants who received other foods as well as breastmilk had:

> 40 per cent fewer episodes of otitis media

This is an important finding, as otitis media can be a cause of deafness and thus a lifelong affliction.

Howie (1990) also found fewer cases of otitis media in breastfed infants in the above mentioned study, although the results were not statistically significant.

The effect of breastfeeding on acute otitis media (AOM) was analyzed in a Swedish study, where 400 children were examined at 2, 6, 10 and 12 months of age. By one year of age, 21 per cent of the children had had at least one episode of AOM (Aniansson, 1994). The frequency was significantly lower in the breastfed children, in every age group, and occurred earlier in children who were weaned before the age of six months of age.

During the examination nasopharyngeal cultures were obtained. Cultures positive for Haemophilus influenzae, Moraxella catarrhalis and Streptococcus pneumoniae were significantly higher in children with AOM. Upper respiratory infection was increased in children with AOM but significantly reduced in the breastfed group.

Necrotising Enterocolitis (NEC)

The cause of NEC has not been conclusively established but may be due to infection (Kleigman, 1979). Lucas et al. (1990) conducted a prospective, multi-centre study of pre-term infants and found that 51 out of 926 infants developed this condition with a mortality rate of 26 per cent. NEC was found to be six to ten times more common if the infant had been fed exclusively with formula milk. Although this condition is rare in babies of more than 30 weeks gestation, it was 20 times more common if the baby received no breastmilk. As most breastmilk banks have been closed, encouraging the mother to provide colostrum and milk for her own baby has become much more important.

Acute appendicitis

Appendicitis is the commonest reason for abdominal surgery in many countries (Heaton, 1987). Knowledge about risk factors for appendicitis is poor. An Italian study (Pisacane et al, 1995) investigated the relationship between breast and formula feeding in 222 children admitted with acute appendicitis and compared them with 222 children randomly selected from 3000 children attending ten randomly selected primary schools.

The study revealed that children who were breastfed for more than four months had a lower incidence of acute appendicitis. This incidence was reduced further if breastfeeding had extended beyond seven months.

It was suggested that the immune components of human milk might be responsible for the decrease in the severity of infection and probably the inflammatory reactions associated with it.

Neurological development

At term the newborn baby's brain weighs about 350g or ten per cent of its total body weight. At the end of the first year it still comprises ten per cent of the total weight, approximately 750g. 60 per cent of the total energy intake during this time is utilized by the brain and much of the energy used to construct the neuronal membrane and myelin comes from the fat of human milk or infant formulas i.e. saturated and polyunsaturated fatty acids (PUFAs) (Cockburn, 1994).

The grey matter, the outer layer of the cerebral cortex, contains 90 per cent of all nerve cells, while the inner white matter is made up of (myelinated) nerve fibres (Toole, 1993). The PUFAs are used for the synthesis of myelin, the substances which insulate cells and aid in the conduction of nerve impulses (Worthington-Roberts, 1993).

Each neurone in the cerebral cortical matter has 10,000 or more discrete areas of membrane responsible for neurotransmission to other nerve cells. These membranes have high concentrations of phospholipids, the long-chain polyunsaturated fatty acids and particularly docosa-hexaenoic acid (DHA) (C22:6n-3) and arachidonic acid (AA) (C20:4n-6) (Cockburn, 1994).

Breastfed infants have a significantly greater concentration of docosahexanoic acid in their cerebral cortex phospholipids than infants fed on infant formulas. Consequently the make-up of the formula-fed infant's brain has been found to be different from that of the breastfed infant, which may be important in neurodevelopmental outcome (Williams, 1994).

A number of studies have investigated differences in cognitive functions between children who were breast or formula fed. To quote just three examples:

1. Morrow-Tlucak et al (1988), measuring cognitive development at two years of age using the Bayley scale, found a 3.7 point advantage in babies breastfed for four months or less and a 9.1 advantage if breastfed for more than four months.

2. Lucas et al (1992) found that premature babies fed with breastmilk had a higher intelligent quotient at the age of seven years.

3. Lanting et al (1994) found a small advantageous effect of breastfeeding in the neurological status in children at nine years of age, in a retrospective study.

Visual acuity

This is also dependent on the development of healthy neural pathways may also be adversely affected by the lack of DHA and AA in infant formulae (Birth, 1993; Uauy, 1990).

Cow's milk allergies and intolerance

Cow's milk allergy (CMA) and cow's milk intolerance (CMI) are mainly problems of infancy and early childhood (Host, 1991). Genetic predisposition and exposure to allergens (mainly cows' milk) are largely responsible for the development of these conditions (Host, 1991). It has also been suggested the infants gut is immature and an incomplete mucosal barrier. Gut permeability therefore allows large molecules to pass into the system setting up immunological responses (Walker, 1987) with the production of serum Immunoglobulin E (IgE). CMA presents mainly with asthma, eczema and allergic rhinitis, while CMI shows itself mainly by an insidious lack of well-being (failure to thrive), persistent restlessness, screaming at intervals and appearing in pain (infantile colic) (Pugh, 1981).

A vast amount of research has been and is being conducted into this problem. A possible adverse effect of feeding babies cow's milk protein is documented in the studies below:

Atherton (1988) also found hypersensitivity to cows' milk to be an important contributory factor in atopic eczema.

Wheezing and allergy were studied by Burr (1993). He found that children who had ever breastfed had a lower incidence of wheeze than those who were fed with cows' milk and soya formula milk. (59 per cent and 74 per cent respectively). In non-atopic breastfed children, the risk of wheeze, after allowing for employment status, sex, passive smoking and overcrowding, was still halved by comparison with those who were artificially fed.

Host (1988) warned against giving breastfed infants an occasional supplement of formula milk because of a possible risk of sensitization. It was suggested that this may be more likely to provoke a subsequent adverse reaction than regular exposure to cow's milk protein.

Jakobsson and Lindberg (1983) found that cows' milk can also affect a small proportion of babies indirectly through the mothers' milk and cause infantile colic. By putting the mothers of susceptible infants on a diet free of cows' milk protein, most infants became symptom free (they subsequently suggested that in about a third of infants with colic, the colic is related to cows' milk in the maternal diet).

The conclusions of another study (Chandra, 1989) were that 'in families with a history of atopic disease mothers should avoid common allergenic foods during lactation'.

Insulin-dependent childhood diabetes

The frequency of childhood insulin dependent diabetes has doubled over the last 15 years. A vast amount of time and effort is spent on research into the cause, prevention and means of arresting the progress of the disease. Karjalainen (1992) found newly diagnosed diabetic children to have a much higher than normal level of IgG anti-BSA. This is the antibody to a cows' milk protein, bovine serum albumin (BSA). By coincidence a section of this milk protein is almost identical to a protein on the islet cells of the pancreas. In genetically predisposed children the anti-BSA antibodies also attack these cells. This auto-immune response is being further researched, but it is possible that five to six per 1000 children are born with this genetic predisposition. Although work is still continuing in this area, the Karjalainen findings have important implications for postnatal care, particularly for the mother who wants to breastfeed. The question must be asked – could one or two bottles of formula milk pre-dispose a baby to insulin-dependent diabetes?

Unless there is a family history of diabetes there is no way of knowing which baby is born with this genetic background (Tarn, 1988).

A ten year, 3000 family study (Alberti, 1993) on childhood diabetes is planned in Scandinavia in which the test group will have no cows' milk for the first nine months of life.

Later benefits of breastfeeding.

Only in the 1980s have studies been published which show health benefits for the breastfeeding mother. Some of the benefits relate to:

Osteoporosis

Osteoporosis is of considerable concern in the elderly woman.

Lindsay (1976) demonstrated in randomized controlled trials that this was mainly due to the lack of oestrogen in menopausal women, which could be improved with oestrogen replacement therapy (Hutchinson, 1979).

It is has been thought that an extra need for calcium during lactation might ultimately result in reduced bone density of the mother, although there is some inconsistency in studies.

Cumming and Klineberg, (1993) have found the reverse to be true. In their study of 311 cases of hip fracture in women over the age of 65 years (living in and around Sydney, Australia) they found that parous women who had not breastfed had twice the risk of hip fracture as nulliparous women and those who had breastfed.

Lactational Amenorrhoea (LAM) - Natural contraception

Aristotle, (384 B.C.- 322 B.C.) whose philosophy was based on empirical observation, noted that 'while women suckle their children, menstruation does not occur according to nature, nor do they conceive.'

This natural contraception has been described recently as the Lactational Amenorrhoea method by researchers at the Institute for Reproductive Health, Georgetown University, Washington (Kennedy, 1989).

Whether the mother is breastfeeding or not, ovulation following childbirth does not occur for 36 days (Perez, 1992). Subsequently, amenorrhoea depends on exclusive breastfeeding (without any supplements), causing the release of high levels of prolactin from the anterior pituitary gland. Prolactin suppresses the pituitary hormones, luteinizing hormone (LH) and follicle stimulating hormone (FSH), which in turn, have an inhibiting influence on the synthesis of ovarian steroids.

Thus the more frequently the baby suckles, the higher the blood levels of prolactin. This in turn is associated with a reduction in the secretion luteinizing hormone and the suppression of ovulation (McNeilly, 1983), although the precise mechanism is not yet understood.

A panel of experts at the 1988 Bellagio Consensus Conference on Lactational Infertility concluded that for amenorrhoeaic women fully (or nearly fully) breastfeeding, 'breastfeeding provides more than 98 per cent protection from pregnancy in the first six months' (Kennedy, 1989).

In order to use the LAM method with confidence, a mother needs to be able to answer 'yes' to all of the following:

• Is your baby less than six months old?

• Are day and night feeds completely unrestricted?

• Is it the case that your baby has no long intervals between feeds?

- Is it the case that your baby is receiving no other food or drink besides breastmilk (apart from token or ritual supplements for religious reasons)?

- Are you amenorrhoeic?

Breast cancer in young women

The United Kingdom Case-Control Study Group (1993) investigating the risk of breast cancer found a correlation between breastfeeding and a reduction in the incidence of this condition in women below the age of 36 years. The risk decreased with increasing duration of breastfeeding, with three months or longer giving the greatest protection.

Breast cancer in menopausal women

In a further study, carried out in Australia, 6,888 women under 75 years newly diagnosed with breast cancer were compared with 11,319 control women without a history of breast cancer (Cumming et. al., 1993). They were interviewed about their reproductive and breastfeeding history. The resulting analysis found a significant trend towards a reduced risk of breast cancer with increasing duration of breastfeeding.

CHAPTER THREE

The Disadvantages of Artificial Feeding

Mass artificial feeding has only been practised in this country for about 50 years. Reliable research about short and long term effects of feeding babies with the adapted milk of another species is only now beginning to be published.

However, throughout the ages some women have either been unwilling or unable to breastfeed (Fildes, 1986).

Since records began, it appears that some mothers found substitutes for their own milk – either another mother's milk, (a wet-nurse) or the milk of another species (Fildes, 1986). In general goat, sheep and cow milk were used, with the latter ultimately becoming the main substitute for human milk.

With the growth of industrialization in the nineteenth century it became increasingly important for women who were factory workers to find a substitute for their own milk.

Hewitt (1958), quoting the evidence given to the 1888 Factory Commission, reported that some married cotton operators returned to work as early as nine days after confinement and most within a fortnight.

Not surprisingly, the replacement of breastmilk with cows' milk, pap made with bread and water sweetened with sugar, or other farinaceous foods, such as oatmeal and sago, had a devastating effect on the health of babies (Hewitt, 1958). Infant diarrhoea became a major health hazard with a considerable rise in infant mortality, which consistently remained above 150 per 1000 live births throughout the nineteenth century.

At around the same time, chemists and medical practitioners began to analyze the composition of human milk and cows' milk and although differences were noted, a number of doctors developed a variety of 'recipes' to produce a more 'scientific' breastmilk substitute (Liebig, 1842). In the mid-nineteenth century the preservation of milk in an evaporated, then condensed, form for infant feeding became possible.

At the beginning of the twentieth century, this was followed by the invention of heated rollers to dry milk and with it the realization of the market potential of baby foods. By the early 1880s numerous products were widely available including those pioneered by James Horlick and Henri Nestle (Apple, 1987).

As the preparation of formula milk became more 'scientific' in the first half of the twentieth century, many people were led to believe that 'formula feeding has become so simple, safe, and uniformly successful that breastfeeding no longer seems worth the bother' (Hill, 1968).

Formula manufacturers know better than anyone how imperfect the substitutes for human milk are. Changes are constantly being made to formula, at least 100 every year (Messenger, 1994). As researchers isolate and identify yet another of breastmilk's components, it is hailed as a new ingredient and added to the formula with the claim that it is now even nearer to breast milk.

Nucleotides, for example, have recently been suggested as co-factors for the growth of bifido bacteria in vitro. The bifido bacteria, present in the gut of the breastfed baby, keep the number of Escherichia Coli under control, whereas bottle fed babies have a larger number of these potential pathogens (Balmer, 1994).

In a study designed to assess the effect of adding nucleotide monophosphate salts to formula feeds, the faecal flora was examined at two weeks of age in:

• 32 babies fed with supplemented whey based formula

• 33 babies with unsupplemented formula

This was compared with the faecal flora of 21 (two week old) breastfed babies, who acted as controls. (Faccal flora were also examined at four weeks and seven weeks of age but with fewer babies in each group).

The greatest differences were found at two weeks of age.

The researchers demonstrated that more babies fed with supplemented formula had their guts colonized with Escherichia coli and more had E coli as the dominant organism in the faecal flora than the unsupplemented group, in whom both bifido bacteria and enterococci were also reduced. This suggests perhaps, that there are other, as yet unknown factors, which are involved in the functioning of nucleotides, and the benefits of breastmilk in this respect cannot be emulated just by adding nucleotides to cows' milk formulae.

Without doubt, babies who were bottle fed 10, 20 or 30 years ago had an inferior milk in comparison to the milk produced today because both knowledge and technology have improved. Just as the artificial milk produced today will be of inferior quality in comparison to the artificial milk in the year 2000.

Formula fed infants

Fomula fed infants are disadvantaged in many ways. Many of the substances found in breastmilk cannot be reproduced. Formula is thus deficient in:

- some nutrient compounds (Epidermal growth factor)

- cells (e.g. leucocytes, macrophages)

- antibodies, anti-bacterial and antiviral factors (e.g. sIgA, IgG, IgM, Lactoferrin)

- hormones (e.g. prolactin, thyroid hormones)

- enzymes (e.g. mammary amylase, milk lipase, lysozyme)

- prostaglandins (to name but a few).

The formula fed infant may be further compromised by:

- the presence of cows' milk or soya proteins

- the possibility of errors during manufacture (Minchin, 1985)

- the addition of new ingredients on an uncertain scientific basis (Stapleton, 1957)

- frequent errors in the preparation of feeds (too much or too little powder in relation to water) which alter the concentration of the feed (Lucas, 1991, 1992)

- the variability of the mineral and trace element content of the water used to re-constitute the formula, before or after sale (Food Chemical News, 1985).

The formula may be inoculated with bacteria and/or other pathogens:

- during the manufacture of milk in the factory and/or

- while preparing the feed at home with unclean utensils and dirty bottles and/or contaminated water

In 1987 Minchin wrote '...only human milk is safe enough for human infants' and '.... contrary to popular belief, even the most sophisticated formula represents a quite unique and unacceptable risk to any child in any place (not just in developing countries) at any time.'

During the 1930s and 1940s concern began to be expressed about the decline in breastfeeding.

Dr J.C. Spence, writing in 1935, attributed this decline in part to the mechanization of breastfeeding and the rules of institutions (including timing feeds and test-weighing of babies) which raised maternal anxiety and increased the difficulty of establishing lactation. He also felt it was in part due to the influence of modern advertising methods on health professionals. He noted that: 'No doctor receives a blotter advertising breastmilk'.

In 1943 the Ministry of Health in a report 'The Breastfeeding of Infants' deplored the increase in the number of babies who were discharged from maternity homes and hospitals *not entirely breastfed*. The percentage of infants not entirely breastfed at the end of fourteen days had risen from 6.5 per cent in 1931 to 12.1 per cent in 1941! The slogan: 'Breastfeeding is best feeding' was coined in this report.

Curiously however, the same Report did not consider the introduction of subsidized National Dried Milk, three years earlier, as a possible contributory factor in the decline of breastfeeding.

In the 1960s and early 1970s local feeding surveys found that far fewer mothers now started to breastfeed and that their numbers rapidly diminished in the first four months of the baby's life. It was during those years that one can say that bottlefeeding became established – the mass, uncontrolled experiment that caused Minchin (1987) such concern. The relatively unmodified cow's milk preparations produced at the time was regarded even by the DHSS as the cause of 'certain hazards to the baby' (Department of Health and Social Security, 1974).

Scowen (1989) described the half and full-cream artificial milks produced in the 1970s as: 'basically cow's milk which had been hygienically prepared in a factory and heat-treated to destroy bacteria'.

From the 1950s onwards, reports in medical journals had been documenting disturbing evidence of an increase in convulsions, (Gittleman and Pincus, 1951; Oppe and Redstone, 1968) brain damage, (McCance and Widdowson, 1957; Macauley and Watson, 1967) and obesity (Taitz, 1971 and Shukla et al. 1972) in artificially fed babies.

Government reports on infant feeding

In 1973 the Chief Medical Officer's Committee on Medical Aspects of Food Policy (COMA) asked the Panel of Child Nutrition to set up a Working Party with the following terms of reference:

> 'to review the present practices of infant feeding and to advise upon these practices.'

The resulting report 'Present Day Practice in Infant Feeding' (1974) highlighted four problems particularly associated with artificial feeding:

Hypernatraemia - due to the high concentration of sodium and potassium in cow's milk

Neonatal tetany - due to the higher concentration of phosphorus

Obesity - due to the tendency of some mothers to make up feeds that were too concentrated

Coeliac Disease - due to the early introduction of cereals.

In its conclusion the Committee stated emphatically that:

> 'satisfactory growth and development after birth is more certain when an infant is fed an adequate volume of breast milk'.

They also made five important recommendations:

i)   that the reconstituted artificial feed ... should approximate to the composition of breastmilk as nearly as practicable (para 5.2.3).

ii)   that the legislation concerning composition, labelling and advertising of milk-based infant foods should be reviewed (para 6.7).

iii) that further research into principles and practice should be made (para 6.5).

vi)   that the patterns of infant feeding should be reviewed on a continuing basis (para 6.6).

v)   that all mothers be encouraged to breastfeed their baby for at least two weeks and preferably for four to six months. (para 5.1.1).

iv)   that health professionals, school children and mothers should be educated about the importance of human milk and breastfeeding (paras 6.2.1 and 2).

As a result of the first recommendation, Professor Oppe was asked by the Panel of Child Nutrition to chair two Working Parties.

Their *first* report, published in 1977, by the DHSS was 'The Composition of Mature Human Milk'

It was based on investigations which analysed breastmilk samples obtained from women in various parts of the country.

The *second* report had been requested by the Food Standards Committee of the Ministry of Agriculture, Fisheries and Food (MAFF) and had the task amongst others of assessing:

•   nutrient composition of infant formula

•   results of feeding trials

•   continued suitability of products

•   the results of further research and advances in knowledge in order to update the compositional guidelines when appropriate

The results were published in 1980 as 'Artificial Feeds for Young Infants', which updated the compositional guidelines for infant formulae. Milk manufacturers had a strong moral obligation to follow the guidelines.

The second recommendation mentioned above had already been introduced in 1976, when the DHSS had issued directions regarding the use of unmodified cow's milk preparations sold for feeding babies below the age of six months (DHSS CNO(76(9). When in 1981, the 34th Assembly of the World Health Organization (WHO) adopted an International Code of Marketing Breastmilk Substitutes, the Government decided that this Code could best be implemented within the United Kingdom by the industry's self regulation.

The Food Manufacturers Federation (FMF) entered into discussions with the DHSS and MAFF and produced The FMF Code of Practice for the Marketing of Infant formula in the United Kingdom, which came into effect in July 1983 together with a complementary Health Circular (HC(83)13).

The European Commission Directive of 14 May 1991 on infant formulae and follow-on formulae obliged the British Government to replace the DHSS guidelines with legislation that was in line with that of the Directive.

The aim was to put into practice the principles and aims of the International Code of Marketing Breastmilk Substitutes adopted by the 34th World Health Assembly, in all countries of the community, bearing in mind their existing particular legal and social situation.

The Directive's acceptance would mean that for the first time the 'compositional and labelling requirements of infant formulae and follow-on formulae for use by infants in good health in the European Economic Community' would become law and a legal framework will be established to set out minimum and maximum permitted levels of named constituents for artificial milks for infants. The regulations would also include marketing and packaging.

On 1st March 1995 the new 'Infant Formula and Follow-on Formula Regulations 1995', Statutory Instruments 1995 No. 77, came into force. The new law includes regulations regarding advertising. It forbids the use of pictures of infants in the labelling of infant formulae or other pictures or text which may idealize the use of the product.

It allows the advertising of infant formulae in publications specializing in baby care and distributed through the health care system, in scientific publications and for the purposes of trade prior to the retail stage.

Such materials must include clear information about the:

•   the benefits and superiority of breastfeeding

•   the possible negative effect on breastfeeding of introducing partial bottlefeeding

•   the difficulty of reversing the decision not to breastfeed.

During the consultation stages 48 agencies, including the British Medical Association, the Royal College of Midwives and the British Paediatric Association supported the United Kingdom proposed total ban of advertising baby milks. However, their efforts were unsuccessful, although the advertising of infant formulae is not allowed in premises where it is sold, nor can free samples be given.

For the third recommendation mentioned above, the DHSS commissioned the Office of Population Censuses and Surveys (OPCS) in 1975 to carry out a survey into infant feeding attitudes and practice (Martin, 1978).

Further surveys have been commissioned every five years since, with a further survey due to be carried out in 1995.

The 1980 and 1985 surveys have formed the basis of 'Present day practice in infant feeding: 1980' (DHSS 1980 and 1983) and 'Present day practice in infant feeding: Third Report' (DHSS, 1988).

In the introduction to chapter three of the Third Report the Committee's recommendation on breastfeeding is clearly stated:

> 'There is no better nutrition for healthy infants, both at term and during the early months'.

Research continues to be published on principles and practice of breastfeeding, as well as the comparison of health outcomes between artificially and breastfed babies.

Some health professionals, who still remain to be convinced of the superiority of breastmilk over formula (Forsyth, 1992), claim that some of the studies which have demonstrated this superiority have been methodologically flawed. The review of 20 of the studies published between 1970 and 1985 (Bauchner, 1986) and on which this claim is largely based, has itself been challenged by Cunningham (1988), but it has received some support from a more recent review of 40 studies published between 1934 and 1990 (Auerbach, 1991).

Nevertheless some of the more recent studies, researching infant health in relation to feeding practices, have taken the criticisms into consideration e.g. of lack of definition of outcome and events, failure to adjust for confounding variables and failure to avoid bias into consideration in their study design.

Studies by Howie (1990) and Lucas (1990) are excellent examples of this.

A review of the current state of the evidence has recently been conducted by the Standing Committee on Nutrition of the British Paediatric Association (1994). It concluded that:

> 'Important differences exist between the composition of breastmilk and artificial formulas. Epidemiological evidence convincingly indicates that breastfed infants are at significantly reduced risk of infection, particularly gastrointestinal infection,

even in industrial societies. Breastfeeding is particularly important for low birthweight infants in whom both reduced mortality...and advantages in cognitive function have been associated with the provision of breastmilk.'

It went on to note the evidence in support of breastmilk's association with increased cognitive development and reduction in IDDM in term infants, and breastfeeding association with a reduction in maternal breast cancer.

Further research remains to be done to enlarge our knowledge of breastmilk and feeding practices. However, health professionals have a responsibility to ensure that their knowledge is as up-to-date as possible. Their clients have the right to receive researched and up-to-date advice, information and support about breastmilk and breastfeeding practice.

Keeping up-to-date with current research findings is not as difficult as it used to be. Several organizations now produce references, outlines or abstracts of current research (e.g. MIDIRS, RCM current awareness, Medline, Cochrane Centre).

CHAPTER FOUR

The Anatomy of the Breasts

A working knowledge of the anatomy of the breast and the physiology of lactation (see Chapters 6 and 13) is essential. It should lead to a reduction in the amount of conflicting advice that is so often given by those who help mothers to establish breastfeeding and/or advise women with breastfeeding problems.

Development of the breasts

Nature begins to prepare for lactation at a very early age. When the embryo is only five weeks old a 'mammary streak' extends on each side from the axilla to the groin. Most of this tissue is reabsorbed but over the chest wall it develops into two breasts, nipples and the surrounding areolae.

Accessory nipples

These together with rudimentary glandular tissue develop occasionally along this streak. Strangely enough they are more common in men than in women (Stanway, 1982). What may appear to be a mole on the line of the 'mammary streak', most commonly in the axillary region, may hide its true nature until a pregnancy ensues. The glandular tissue behind the mole begins to grow with the stimulation of pregnancy hormones. This very rarely causes problems but may become uncomfortable and even painful when the milk comes in. However as these rudimentary breasts are not stimulated they soon return to their pre-pregnancy size. Very rarely they may have to be removed surgically.

The newborn's breasts

Following birth the mammary tissue of the breasts of a newborn baby (of either sex) may respond to the maternal hormones oestrogen and progesterone, and swell temporarily, producing a fluid sometimes referred to as witches' milk. These swellings resolve without treatment within a week (Worthington-Roberts, 1993).

No further changes occur until two to three years before the onset of the menarche, when the ovaries begin to be active (Riordan, 1993). The breasts then begin to grow under the influence of ovarian oestrogen and progesterone.

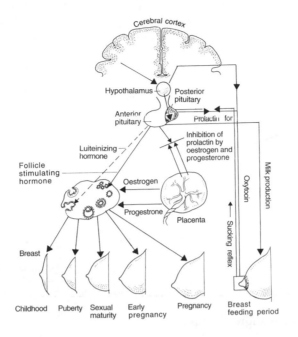

The hormonal effect on the breasts

The gross structure of the breasts

Covered by skin, the base of the breasts lie in the superficial fascia of the pectoralis muscle between the second and sixth rib and from the lateral margin of the sternum to the mid-axillary line. They are separated from the deep fascia covering the muscle by an area of loose connective tissue (Snell, 1995).

The base of the breasts is roughly circular in shape with an extension towards the axilla, 'the axillary tail of Spence' (Lawrence, 1994).

The size and shape of the breasts differ from woman to woman and depend on the amount of adipose tissue laid down during puberty. This covers and is distributed around the glandular tissue.

The *glandular tissue* is arranged in 15-20 lobes, like segments of an orange, pointing towards the centre, the nipple. The lobes are separated from each other by septa of fibrous tissue. The septa in the upper part of the breast are well developed extend from the skin to the deep fascia. They serve as suspensory ligaments.

The minute structure of the breast

Each *glandular lobe* divides into *smaller lobes* and *lobules*, terminating in groups of *alveoli*, which are lined with milk secreting cells, the *cells of Acini*. Surrounding the alveoli is a network of *blood vessels* and *myo-epithelial muscle fibres*. The latter are sensitive to oxytocin.

27

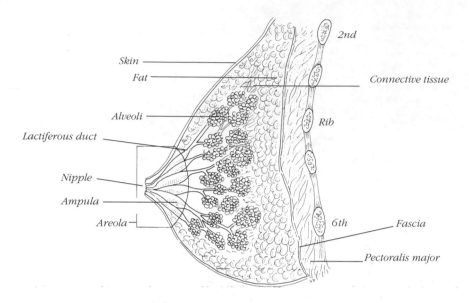

Schematic section through a breast

The alveoli open into *minute ductules*, which join to form larger ducts and become the *lactiferous ducts*. Beneath the areola the ducts are thought to widen into the distensible *lactiferous sinuses or ampullae* in which milk may collect. These sinuses are palpable in a lactating women. The ducts narrow again as they pass through the *nipple* to open on its surface.

The *nipple*, situated just below the centre of the breast, is pink or light brown in colour and contains two types of muscle fibres:

- circular, sphincter-like muscle fibres (surrounding the ducts)

- erectile, erogenous muscle fibres lying alongside the ducts. These respond to touch, cold and sexual stimulation.

Most commonly nipples are projectile. However, some ten per cent of pregnant women who intend to breastfeed have inverted or non protractile nipples (Alexander, 1992).

The *areola* is a pink or light brown circular area of variable size. It surrounds the nipple. The 12 - 18 minute projections on its surface are the *Montgomery's tubercles*, a type of sebaceous gland. They are said to lubricate the areola and nipple during pregnancy and lactation. Both the nipple and areola are well supplied with nerve endings.

Blood supply

The breasts receive *arterial blood* from three different sources:

• the upper intercostal arteries, branching from the aorta

• the internal mammary artery, arising from the subclavian artery on the right and aorta on the left

• the external mammary artery, a branch from the lateral thoracic artery.

Venous drainage is via the internal mammary and axillary veins. Anastomosis of the vessels around the nipple becomes visible as the marbling appearance of the breasts in pregnancy and early lactation.

Lymphatic drainage

A large lymphatic network drains mainly into the axillary and para-sternal, pectoral and liver glands or nodes. The lymphatic connection between the right and left breast is of particular concern in breast cancer.

The nerves of the breast

Branches from the fourth, fifth and sixth thoracic nerves supply the sensory innervation of the breasts. The nipple and areola in particular are richly endowed with sensory nerve fibres.

The breasts in pregnancy

The breast undergo their final stage of growth during pregnancy. Under the influence of *oestrogen* the ducts increase in size and length, while progesterone stimulates the proliferation of the glandular tissue, thus increasing the size of the breasts.

A sensation of tingling, fullness and heaviness of the breasts are often the first signs of pregnancy.

Small amounts of prolactin, secreted by the anterior pituitary gland stimulates the Acini cells to secrete protein, carbohydrate and fat, while the duct system secretes fluids and electrolytes-*colostrum*. A few drops can be expressed from approximately 16 weeks. Actual milk production is inhibited by the high levels of progesterone and oestrogen.

During pregnancy the areola darkens, perhaps to enable the baby to focus on it in his/her 'search' for the nipple.

Some women develop a *secondary areola* in the latter half of pregnancy, as a paler brown area around the primary areola.

Pregnancy may cause the nipple to become slightly larger.

CHAPTER FIVE

Looking After the Breasts in Pregnancy

All women are encouraged to practice breast self-examination for disease detection. When they become pregnant, they will find that the changes in the consistency of the breasts will be palpable very early on. They become lumpy and tender and as the glandular tissue increases they become heavier and larger.

Breast examination

At the first antenatal examination, at home or in the booking clinic, the breasts are examined for two purposes – for medical reasons and with a view to breastfeeding. Any special aspects are noted and recorded. If conditions such as cysts, dimpling of the skin or lumps are detected, the relevant investigations and treatment can be initiated.

In relation to breastfeeding any scars and surgery would be relevant (see below). With the exception of a history of breast cancer, when breastfeeding is contra-indicated, (Lawrence, 1994) an individual assessment in relation to previous surgery will determine whether breastfeeding should be encouraged or not.

The most common reasons for breast scars are:

•   cosmetic surgery to enlarge or reduce breast size
•   a previous breast abscess, biopsy, lumpectomy or rarely a mastectomy
•   scalding or burns

It should be noted whether the nipples are flat or inverted. Unless the woman wishes to discuss her nipples in particular or breastfeeding in general, it should be left to a later stage. It is not only unnecessary in early pregnancy, it may even be counter-productive (Alexander, 1990; RCM, 1991).

The only advice/information that might be useful at this stage is that the dried secretion sometimes found on the nipple is a little colostrum which has oozed out. This can be removed with water only. Soap should be avoided if possible to prevent washing off the natural lubrication of the areola from the Montgomery's tubercles.

Care of the breasts

'Education, information and reassurance for the pregnant women' are considered by Hall to be one of the three major components of antenatal care (Hall, 1984). However there is little research based evidence to support the advice on breast care that may be given to mothers in pregnancy. Alexander (1990) considers that 'women should not be given the impression that it is essential to wear a bra... or...that it conveys any physical benefit. This matter should be governed by the woman's wishes and comfort'.

The Stanways (1983) were of the opinion that 'If the shape of [the] breasts is altered at all, it will probably be due to the pregnancy, and not breastfeeding'.

However they felt that if the breasts were not well supported as they grew in pregnancy and later when the milk comes in, they might lose their shape regardless of whether they were used to feed a baby. The only support in the breasts is the fibrous connective tissue framework within the breasts. This is not elastic and therefore will not recoil if it has been stretched, when the breasts eventually return to their non pregnant size. It might be supposed that a woman with large breasts is also likely to be more comfortable with a well-supporting bra to prevent the breasts from dragging.

The decision to breastfeed

93 per cent of the women who took part in the 1990 Infant Feeding Survey had decided how they would feed their baby before they ever became pregnant (White, 1992). 88 per cent (n-5372) of the mothers in the survey had been asked about their feeding intention and 45 per cent of these mothers had also had some discussion about feeding method. This discussion seemed to have had no influence on the initial feeding intention (The survey did not ask about the timing of this discussion).

Early doubts about breastfeeding success

Many women who have decided to breastfeed their babies are concerned about their ability to do so.

When a woman is asked by the midwife about her feeding intention, a common reply is: 'I'm going to *try and breastfeed*'. This guarded response is not surprising as many women will have a friend, relation or acquaintance who was one of the many mothers who, overcome by problems, gave up breastfeeding earlier than she had intended (20 per cent by the end of week two) (White, 1992).

She may also have read articles on breastfeeding in women's, parents' and baby magazines, which largely deal with breast feeding problems and difficulties.

Nipple preparation for breastfeeding

The erectile structure of the nipple becomes evident if it is touched or if cold water is applied. In pregnancy this protraction becomes more pronounced. In about 10 per cent of women the nipples are 'hidden' or inverted and non-protractile (Alexander, 1992).

Numerous studies have reported a variety of methods for nipple preparation. What has underpinned those reviewed by Alexander (1990) is the mistaken notion that it is necessary to toughen the nipple in order to breastfeed successfully and that breastfeeding is all about nipples.

Difficulties in latching the baby to the breast are frequently blamed on 'poor nipples' rather than the lack of support and skill in helping a mother to achieve good positioning of the baby at the breast. Perhaps the problem of conflicting advice given for breastfeeding problems also begins in the antenatal period.

Having reviewed the research on nipple preparation prior to conducting her own randomized controlled trial, Alexander (1990) concluded that,

> 'nipple protractibility should be assessed late in the second or early in the third trimester, the results being thoroughly discussed with the woman. If she is found to have an inverted or non-protractile nipple she should then choose whether she wishes to have treatment and if so, what. No other preparation is required and no soap should be used when washing the nipple, as it destroys the natural protective lubrication.'

In 1943 a report from the Ministry of Health deplored the 'diversity of teaching' found in standard textbooks on the preparation of the breasts during pregnancy and suggested that 'it (is) possible that... too much stress on preparation of the breasts may alarm and discourage (a woman) to such an extent that she will refuse even to initiate breastfeeding'.

Alexander's research reaffirmed this suggestion 17 of the 128 pregnant women who had decided to breastfeed and who were approached to take part in her study on the treatment of non-protractile and inverted nipples subsequently decided against breastfeeding. Her conclusion was that '...the process of screening pregnant women for nipple problems may act as a disincentive to successful breastfeeding for women with such problems' (Alexander, 1992).

Hoffman's exercises and breast shells

The two methods of nipple preparation Alexander investigated were:

- the use of breast shells
- Hoffman's exercises

These were used both singly and in combination and compared with a group who received no nipple preparation. The main outcome measure was the success of breastfeeding reported by postnatal questionnaire six weeks postnatally. The study found that neither shells nor exercises conferred any benefit. On balance shells appeared to do more harm than good. The value of Hoffman's exercises was more open to question, although her trial showed no difference between the group allocated exercises and the group allocated no exercises, the size of her trial meant that a clinically useful effect could not be ruled out.

For that reason a much larger study investigating the same methods of nipple preparation, the MAIN (Multicentre Randomized Controlled Trial of Alternative Treatments for Inverted and Non-protractile Nipples in Pregnancy) trial was carried out in conjunction with the National Perinatal Epidemiology Unit in Oxford.

This study confirmed Alexander's findings that neither method conferred any benefit and ruled out the hypothesized benefit of exercises. The authors concluded:

> '...there is no basis for recommending the use of either Hoffman's nipple stretching exercises or breast shells as antenatal preparation for women with inverted and non-protractile nipples who wish to breastfeed. Given the lack of evidence to support this and other antenatal preparations there are no grounds for midwives to continue routine breast examination for this purpose.' (The MAIN trial Collaborative Group, 1994).

Although the current recommendation is thus that the nipples should not be examined, there will always be some women who want to prepare their nipples for breastfeeding. They should understand that nipples cannot be toughened but they can become accustomed to being handled.

A partner's help

If it is acceptable to the woman and her partner, nipple sucking can become part of love play. Hewat and Ellis (1987) found that oral stimulation of the nipple correlated significantly with less postnatal nipple trauma.

There is a theoretical risk that stimulation of the nipple may cause the posterior pituitary gland to release oxytocin, thus initiating uterine contractions. No such effect was detected in the MAIN trial amongst those women allocated to use Hoffman's exercises, but the numbers were small and such an effect cannot be ruled out. Any preparation might thus be inadvisable if the woman has previously experienced a premature birth or if during the current pregnancy has threatened to go into early labour.

Nipple rolling

Nipple rolling was not evaluated in the MAIN trial but has been investigated by other researchers and reviewed by Alexander (1990). There is no evidence that it is of benefit.

The 'niplette'

In 1992 a Consultant Plastic Surgeon who had been treating inverted nipples for *cosmetic reasons* with surgery developed a device for their correction called a 'niplette'

(McGeorge, 1993). The device consists of a thimble-shaped plastic mould with a sealing flange attached to a valve and syringe.

The 'niplette' is designed to be placed over the nipple area and the syringe drawn out gently. The valve creates a vacuum and gentle suction draws the nipple out into the thimble, thereby lengthening the lactiferous sinuses. Once the 'niplette' is attached it can be worn under loose clothing for up to 24 hours a day.

A report on the use of this device by 22 women, six of them pregnant, noted that sustained correction was achieved by all but one of the women and took between one to three months (McGeorge, 1993). A further eight pregnant women were said to have used the device after the original report was submitted for publication and all fourteen of them were said to be breastfeeding successfully, six of them after failing to do so with previous children.

During the treatment, two of the patients had slight bleeding from their nipples, one pulled too hard, the other, using the device late in pregnancy, experienced occasional minor bleeds.

It needs to be borne in mind that 45 per cent of the women with inverted nipples who were recruited to the MAIN trial and received no treatment whatsoever, were reported to be successfully breastfeeding at six weeks. The dangers of extrapolating the use of a device designed as a substitute for the (cosmetic) surgical correction of inverted nipples in non-pregnant women, to use in the antenatal period, have been highlighted (Inch and Fisher, 1993; McCandish, 1993).

A properly conducted, randomized controlled trial needs to be carried out before midwives will be in a position to judge whether it does more good than harm.

Conclusion

There is currently no evidence that any form of nipple treatment or preparation contributes in anyway to successful breastfeeding. Midwives can reassure women with inverted nipples that their chances of being able to breastfeeding successfully are no less than that of women in the general population as sampled by OPCS (White, 1992).

CHAPTER SIX

The Physiology of Lactation

The term lactation includes both the production of milk and the secretion of milk. These functions become established as a result of two *neuro-hormonal reflex actions*.

Lactogenesis - the initiation of lactation

Following the delivery of the placenta, the levels of oestrogen and progesterone in the blood begin to fall. This allows the already high levels of prolactin to act on the breast and begin milk production, whether the breasts are stimulated by a suckling baby or not. If the mother has decided not to breastfeed, the prolactin levels will gradually fall to the non-pregnant levels within a fortnight and the milk will gradually be reabsorbed (Lawrence, 1994). Unrestricted early suckling (demand feeding) however, increases the levels of circulating prolactin and milk will 'come in' sooner than it would if the baby were fed on a restricted schedule (Carvalho, 1983; Salaryia, 1978).

The lactation reflexes

These are neuro-hormonal reflexes and are mediated via the hypothalamus.

The let-down or milk ejection reflex

The touch of the baby's lips on the nipple and areola, together with the sensation of suckling, sends nerve messages via the hypothalamus to the *posterior pituitary gland* and *oxytocin* is released into the bloodstream. This initiates the *let down or milk ejection reflex*. That is to say the myo-epithelial cells, sensitive to oxytocin, respond by contracting and squeezing the milk in the alveoli into the ducts towards the nipple and the milk starts to flow. At first this reflex is unconditioned and requires a physical stimulus. Eventually it becomes a conditioned reflex – for instance just thinking about her baby or hearing a baby cry can start the breasts to leak.

Once it has become conditioned, the reflex can be affected by physical stress, such as painful breasts or nipples, emotional stress such as embarrassment, lack of confidence, worry or severe shock (Newton, 1948).

The hypothalamus being the seat of emotions suppresses the release of oxytocin from the posterior pituitary gland. However, this inhibition is both partial and temporary.

The milk-production or prolactin reflex

As the breast is cleared of the accumulated colostrum or milk by the baby's suckling, a second nerve signal reaches the hypothalamus and effects the *release of prolactin* from the *anterior pituitary gland*.

Clearing the breast is thus the stimulus for the production of a good milk supply (Carvalho, 1983; Salaryia, 1978).

In addition, the milk in the breast contains an inhibitory factor for milk production (Pcakcr, 1987). If this is allowed to build up in the breast this will also reduce milk production (Prentice, 1989).

Thus the more often a breast is 'emptied' the more milk is produced whereas a reduction in the number of times a baby is put to the breast will decrease the milk supply.

Establishment and maintenance of lactation

Nature is generous and most mothers have enough milk in the early days to feed two babies. Thus the mother of a single baby may find that she produces more than her baby needs. In consequence, many babies are satisfied suckling from just one breast at a feed.

Where this is the case, stimulating each breast only every other feed will reduce and regulate the milk supply, so that eventually the baby will probably need to suckle on both breasts at each feed.

It takes between six to eight weeks for breastfeeding to become established, during which time the breasts 'learn' to produce the amount of milk the baby needs at each feed. By this stage the supply of milk is regulated by the amount the baby takes at each feed rather than by prolactin release (Daly, 1993).

As the lactation period progresses the mother may be more aware of the let-down reflex coming into operation. Many mothers feel a warm and tingling sensation within the breasts as the milk is released. As the baby feeds this process may be repeated.

The vast majority of mothers can provide all the milk their baby needs to thrive. The problem of milk insufficiency is discussed in a later chapter.

CHAPTER SEVEN

The Nature of Suckling

Suckling has been called a 'high-frequency micro-rhythm', an apparently simple activity which is organized in complex time sequences (Schaffer, 1977). Whereas the mother has to learn how to breastfeed her baby, the baby 'knows' how to co-ordinate the sequence of steps which embrace the total feeding mechanism. This complex inborn skill of the newborn baby ensures its survival.

The reflexes

This instinctive knowledge incorporate three well known reflexes.

The rooting reflex - searching for the breast with his mouth wide open, the tongue moves over the lip (the latter is sometimes called the extrusion reflex). He then scoops up the nipple and breast tissue, containing the ampullae, into his mouth shaping it into a teat. This reflex can be elicited by stroking the baby's cheek or by touching the lips with the nipple.

The suckling reflex - this is stimulated when the tip of the nipple reaches the back of the mouth and comprises two simultaneous movements:

• the up and down movement of the lower jaw

• the muscular movement of the tongue as it compresses the teat against the hard palate in a wave-like motion.

This propels the milk collected in the ampullae along the ducts to the tip of the nipple at the back of the baby's mouth.

The swallowing reflex - as the milk reaches the oropharynx, the soft palate rises and shuts off the nasopharynx. At the same time, the larynx is raised and closes the trachea and the milk is pushed into the oesophagus.

Woolridge (1986) has described and illustrated these dynamic events and relationships and drawn attention to their relevance for adequate milk transfer and the prevention of sore nipples.

Feeding at the breast

The rhythmical suckling pattern of the well positioned baby is likely to be governed by the rate of milk flow, vigour and the need for milk (Wolff, 1967).

At the beginning of each feed a typical pattern follows the latching-on process:

• It starts with a short period of non-nutritive sucking quick - shallow sucks without swallowing - which stimulates the let-down reflex. At first this can take up to a minute or so before the milk begins to flow. Later, just thinking about feeding or hearing the baby cry can initiate the let-down reflex.

• When the milk begins to flow the suckling pattern changes to a period of continuous, slow, deep suckling, followed by a pause.

This pattern repeats itself, until

• the periods of suckling gradually become shorter and the pauses longer

• eventually the baby lets go of the breast spontaneously which signals that the baby has had enough.

If the baby, having had time to recover from the first breast, or perhaps having burped, shows signs that he is still hungry, the same pattern will repeat itself at the second breast.

Sometimes the baby will come off the first side after just a few minutes and burp. In this case he should be offered the same side again.

Nipple sucking at the breast

The pattern described above does not occur with the baby who is not well positioned at the breast and is nipple-sucking. The pattern of shallow *sucking* does not change into the deep slow *suckling* and swallowing rhythm and is an indication that the baby needs to be re-positioned. Righard et al (1992) suggested that a change from a correct *suckling* technique to shallow *sucking* may be due to the introduction of the occasional bottle feed. He suggests that the infant has had to cope with two different techniques, suckling and sucking and finds this difficult. A common expression used in America for this is 'nipple-confusion'.

There is, however, no evidence to support this suggestion and many babies who have had to receive their mothers' milk by bottle, for some reason, have no difficulty in adapting to the breast.

Nipple confusion versus aversion behaviour

It may be that a baby who has had a repeatedly frustrating and/or traumatic time at the breast and who is then offered a bottle may subsequently prefer to take a bottle, because it does not carry with it the negative associations of the breast (Woolridge 1993). This is not the same as being unable to distinguish between or cope with two different methods of feeding.

It is probable that the baby is using the same basic technique for both the breast and the bottle but that the rippling action of the tongue, seen at the breast, appears as a more up-and-down movement of the jaw with a bottle, because the bottle teat is much harder and less flexible.

CHAPTER EIGHT

Starting Breastfeeding

Grantly Dick Read, an astute observer of mothers, wrote about breastfeeding in his book *Childbirth Without Fear* (1954). He said:

> 'The newborn baby has only three demands: warmth in the arms of its mother, food from her breast and security in the knowledge of her presence. Breastfeeding satisfies all three'.

In other words breastfeeding fulfils the newborn's physiological, nutritional, psychological and emotional needs.

Helping a mother with the first feed

A peaceful, unhurried atmosphere serves to relax the mother. Not all babies want to suckle immediately, especially if the birth has been tranquil (Henschel, 1980 unpublished pilot study). While the baby takes time to adjust to his new world, the mother can enjoy, explore and cuddle her baby. If the baby has to be separated from his mother for any reason, it does not mean that breastfeeding cannot succeed. (After all, even women who adopt a baby can stimulate a milk supply by repeated frequent suckling!)

A skilful, sensitive helper, ideally the midwife who cared for the mother in labour, should know whether the mother expects hands-on help or wants to put the baby to the breast by herself. But the mother should be offered the opportunity as soon as the baby searches for the nipple (e.g. as soon as the rooting reflex becomes evident).

The need to suckle is common to all mammalian young. Hardly born, many are able to stagger to their feet and within a few minutes are able to find the mother's teat to suckle.

Are the human newborn really so different? I don't think so. A recent video recording made in Sweden demonstrated that when the baby is left on the mother's abdomen after birth, it will crawl towards the breast, search and find the nipple and latch on (Widstrom, 1994).

Many midwives will have witnessed the birth of a baby whose mother laboured without analgesia and gave birth in an upright position - standing, on her knees or squatting. This is the ideal position for her to welcome her baby, hold it against her naked skin and suckle it, when it begins to root or search for the nipple.

Michel Odent, the French obstetrician, brought this to our attention in his book *Birth Reborn* (1984). In his practice he ensures that the environment is warm, quiet and with dim lighting. Mother and baby are not disturbed in their first minutes together so that they can communicate with each other.

He writes:

> 'Not only do infants know how to look for and find their mothers' breasts almost immediately, but mothers also know what to do - they act instinctively to help their baby nurse.

> ... Sometimes even a mother who had no intention of breastfeeding will start to nurse her baby right after birth, not remembering until some hours later that she had planned to bottlefeed'.

A number of researchers have found that satisfying this early urge to suckle positively influences the success and the duration of breastfeeding (Klaus et al, 1982; Sosa et al, 1978; De Chateau, 1977; Salariya, 1978).

If most babies are ready to suckle after the birth, what of the mothers? Are *they* ready to suckle their baby? Do *we,* the carers, provide a background environment that is conducive to breastfeeding, so that they *are* ready?

If we believe breastfeeding matters, we ought to give serious thought to creating the right ambience so that this early suckling is successful. Again, Grantly Dick Read recognized this in 1954 when he wrote:

> 'The ability of the mother to feed her baby at the breast is commensurate with her ability to give birth to the child without assistance and interference. The mothers who witness the arrival of the baby and experience relief, joy, achievement and pride that are the natural accompaniment to the birth of the child, invariably desire to feed their babies, and not infrequently, are able to do so efficiently. We cannot disassociate breastfeeding from the manner of birth... This could be put in another way: that the nearer the birth of a child to the normal physiological function, so much more likely is the continuity of the natural sequence of events of human reproduction maintained'.

Effect of labour ward practices on breastfeeding

However, the birth-feed interval is not the only aspect that affects breastfeeding. Earlier circumstances surrounding labour also influence its success.

Kroeger (1993) presented a thought provoking paper at the 23rd International Congress of the International Confederation of Midwives and suggested an eleventh step to be added to the 'Ten Steps to Successful Breastfeeding', a global project initiated by WHO/UNICEF in 1992 (see Appendix II).

She considered the eleventh step to be:

> 'Labor and delivery practices must promote a climate where early interaction is optimized'

She reiterated the observations made by Grantly Dick Read, that many common labour ward practices do *not* provide a setting for positive, early interaction between mother and baby.

For example, it is still not uncommon to find that the mother has:

- adopted a recumbent position throughout most of the labour

- being prevented from drinking nourishing fluids

- received medication with analgesia

- been subjected to electronic fetal monitoring, episiotomy, instrumental delivery or caesarean section.

Maternal analgesia and breastfeeding

Pethidine, a narcotic analgesic, the most common form of pain relief used in labour, causes as a side effect, central nervous system depression. Once the baby is born it is therefore not surprising that a mother who was given Pethidine as an analgesic is only too ready to sink into drowsiness, now no longer interrupted by contractions.

Putting the baby to the breast at this stage is an effort for her and she may welcome a delay.

An increasing number of studies have documented the effect of Pethidine also on the baby, causing neuro-behavioral changes, e.g. less eye-to-eye contact (Stechler, 1964) and a reduced response to sound (Brackbill, 1974).

Maternal analgesia also affects the sucking behaviour of both artificially and breastfed babies adversely (Hodgkinson, 1978; Matthews, 1989; Rajan, 1993). To compound this situation, Pethidine is excreted into the breastmilk for at least two days post-partum.

T.B. Brazelton in 'Maternal-Infant Bonding' comments:

> 'Certainly a depressed infant is less likely to be responsive on initial contact or during feeding situations, and he becomes less stimulated and responsive to a mother who is trying hard to mobilize herself to attach to her new infant' (Klaus and Kennell, 1976).

Righard (1990) throws further light on the feeding behaviour of 72 babies in a non-randomized study of the effect of delivery room routines on suckling behaviour during the first two hours following birth.

One group of babies (n=38) were left undisturbed on their mothers' abdomen, while the control group (n=34) received conventional treatment with the baby left on their mother's abdomen for 20 minutes and then separated for measuring and dressing, before being returned to the mother.

The observations found that the babies in the undisturbed group latched themselves on correctly without help (24/38) while the babies of the separation group had more difficulties, even with help (7/34).

However, separation and maternal use of Pethidine in labour resulted in the most negative outcome and none in this group of babies breastfed successfully during the first two hours following delivery (40/72).

These observers were also confirmed in a study by Rajan (1994), who found that certain groups of mothers are frequently not ready to suckle their baby after birth. Using information derived from the 'UK National Birthday Trust Fund Pain Relief in Labour' (1990), and based on a sample of 1035, she confirmed that the more obstetric intervention there is during labour and delivery, the less likely is a woman to be breastfeeding at six weeks.

This applied particularly if:

- pethidine was used in labour

- the membranes were ruptured artificially

- labour was induced

- oxytocin was used to accelerate the second stage of labour

- the mother had a violent and exhausting birth and assisted delivery.

Clearly, interventions are sometimes necessary. However, as we now know the deleterious effect of the above on breastfeeding, Rajan suggests that the recommendations made by Murray et al (1981) should be adopted. These proposed that efforts should be made to counteract and overcome initial problems such as exhaustion, drowsiness, pain and/or an unresponsive baby.

This is the prime responsibility of the midwife. In fact, satisfaction with midwifery care was found to be an important factor in contributing to breastfeeding success in Rajan's study.

Thus for a mother, the experience of the first feed is special and the outcome will colour the feelings she brings to subsequent feeds. A good suckling experience will leave her with a glow of self confidence.

Routine care after birth

When the baby is offered the breast, some time after birth, it happens not infrequently that the baby is unresponsive and appears not to want to suckle. Could this be due to something other than pethidine or other drugs used in labour?

Did the baby root and show an interest earlier on, and were those special moments when he wanted to suckle, lost? We need to look at our routine care in the labour ward.

What *does* generally happen during those first two hours following the birth of a baby? The priorities of care given during the early hours following birth are concerned with many practical matters.

For the mother this means:

- the third stage of labour has to be completed

- the perineum may have to be repaired

- the mother has to be made comfortable/washed

- observations have to be carried out and documented.

The baby may be separated from the mother for:

- resuscitation

- a general examination

- washing, weighing and dressing.

A midwife's responsibility also demands that she:

- completes the necessary records

- cares for other mothers in labour.

Breastfeeding has to compete with this list of activities.

Furthermore, the mother may feel that she needs permission to put the baby to the breast or find that the help that she feels she needs is not available because the midwife is engaged elsewhere.

The initial breastfeed on the postnatal ward

In general mother and baby are transferred as quickly as possible to the postnatal ward, in order to free the labour ward bed. If she arrives on the postnatal ward during the night, the mother is often encouraged to sleep. If she arrives during the day, the first feed is not always given priority, and because of liberal visiting hours, visitors may already be waiting to see the new arrival.

Changing established practices is not easy and different circumstances in individual maternity units call for a variety of solutions to create the optimum environment to give breastfeeding a successful beginning (and implement Kroeger's eleventh step). However, as research has shown that early suckling and contact of the mother with her baby increases the success of breastfeeding (De Chateau, 1977; Inch and Garforth, 1998; Lindenberg 1990) it behoves us to find time and look for practical and possible solutions to achieve this as often as possible.

CHAPTER NINE

The Skill of Breastfeeding

Correct positioning is the secret of successful breastfeeding. However well meaning the advice, help and support given to the breastfeeding mother, unless the positioning of the baby at the breast is correct, the problems created are highly likely to lead to the discontinuation of breastfeeding.

The problems are:

• insufficient milk

• painful breasts or nipples

• breastfeeding takes too long/tiring.
(Martin, 1988; White, 1992)

In some cultures these problems do not seem to exist. Breastfeeding is a natural part of life and of growing up and is not hidden behind closed doors. Breastfeeding is easy and natural. So, for instance, young girls absorb the simple knowledge of how to hold the baby for breastfeeding quite unconsciously, as they see breastfeeding all around them, often their own mothers, sisters or friends (Toothill, 1995). In our culture new mothers have generally only seen babies being bottlefed so they tend to hold the baby in the crook of their arm and lying on its back when trying to breastfeed.

Positioning a baby at the breast is therefore a *skill to be learned*, just as, for example, one needs to learn the individual movements of a dance or how to use the hands to shape the clay on a potter's wheel. Every skill starts with a number of individual steps, which eventually flow into each other to become an effortless movement.

The role of the midwife

Of prime importance is an unhurried and calm environment where the mother looks forward to the first suckling. This goes a long way towards achieving success.

Next, the midwife must be sensitive to the needs of the individual mother. The help given will vary. It can take the form of:

• hands-on help

- talking the mother through the positioning skill so that she manages to put the baby to the breast herself

- leaving her to manage by herself, if that is her preference.

In which ever way the baby achieves correct positioning the midwife should share in the joy of her success. Sharing in this achievement will raise the mother's self-confidence and self esteem, so often lacking in her vulnerable new role. If the mother does not want any help, this does not make the midwife superfluous, nor does it denigrate her role.

On the other hand, if the mother does need active help, the midwife now needs to use her skills to help and encourage her in such a way that the mother's confidence in her ability to do it herself in the future is not undermined.

Preparation of the mother

Breastfeeding should be considered a rest time! In the first few days this may not be a priority in the mother's mind, as she focuses on the baby. But because her concentration should not be disturbed by discomfort or pain, the midwife should ensure she can relax in the position of her choice, sitting up or lying on her side.

It takes some experimenting to find the optimum position for an individual mother, but whether sitting on a chair or in bed her position should be upright with good back support. In hospital a number of ways can be suggested.

Sitting:

- up in bed with a backrest and sufficient pillows to ensure that she is not leaning back (This is difficult if the mother's legs are stretched out in front of her).

- on the edge of the bed with the feet on a chair or footstool (or on the floor, if the bed can be lowered).

- 'taylor' position on the bed or the floor.

- on an upright chair.

If using the latter, ideally the height of a chair should enable the mother to have her feet flat on the floor, with her lap almost flat; i.e. knees slightly raised. A low foot stool or a couple of telephone directories under the foot of the side from which the baby is going to feed helps to support the baby. This would be a better way than crossing legs, which can stem the blood flow and lead to stasis. Depending on the size of the baby and the mother's breasts, a pillow on her lap can be helpful to bring the baby up to the right level.

Sometimes the sitting position may be difficult or painful e.g. following a caesarean section, an epidural or if she has a sore perineum. Lying on her side may be a good alternative.

The breasts should be free of clothing and because breastfeeding often makes the mother thirsty, a drink should be at hand.

Preparation of the baby

If the baby is calm and relaxed it helps to get the feed started well. On the other hand, if the baby is fractious it may be easier for someone other than the mother to calm the baby. Because of his acute sense of smell, he will recognize his mother's scent and the urge to feed will be increased (Klaus and Kennell, 1982).

In the beginning it may be helpful to swaddle the baby, who is also learning, so that in the eagerness to suckle the hands don't compete with the breast.

Beginning to breastfeed

There is no *one* right way to hold a baby to breastfeed successfully. Once a mother understands the underlying principles of good attachment, she will see that they are the same whatever the position. The position she uses should be one in which she can most easily put the underlying principles into practice. Some of the more common variations are detailed below:

Lying comfortably and close to the mother, the baby's body and head should be in one line, facing her and the head should be slightly higher than the bottom.

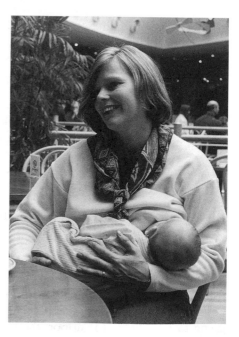

The baby's head should lie on her forearm, rather than in the crook of her elbow, with the nose/upper lip opposite the nipple. At the same time the head should be slightly extended so that the chin is nearer to the breast than is the nose.

Often called the 'Madonna' hold

The baby lies across the lap as before. The mother supports the baby's head and shoulders with the hand that is opposite the breast being fed from, in such a way that his head is free to extend slightly as he is brought to the breast. Her index finger and her thumb support the baby's head as he is moved to the breast. Alternatively, she may make a 'platform' with all of her fingers to support the side of the baby's head.

Her thumb will then be behind the baby's head, but it will exert no pressure. Care should be taken to keep the head slightly extended. If the head is flexed as the baby is moved to the breast he cannot open his mouth properly and consequently can not latch on well.

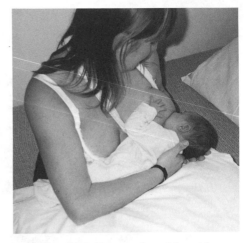

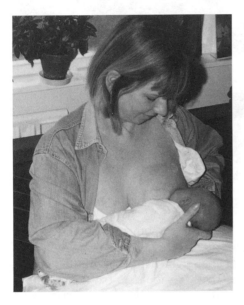

Holding the baby comfortably with both hands

The baby should be placed in such a way that the nose, not the mouth, is in line with the nipple before the feed begins, and so that he comes up to the breast from below i.e. his upper eye could make contact with his mother's.

Holding the baby with one arm and the breast with the other

Baby's body is held under the arm. A chair with an arm rest may be useful for this position. Alternatively the mother could sit on the side of the bed, with her feet over the edge (and supported, see above) with pillows beside her. The baby is tucked under the mother's arm, his body either curled around her body or stretching backwards. The hand of the same side supports the head and shoulders and the opposite hand the breast. This can be adapted to feed both twins at the same time but of course the breasts cannot be supported.

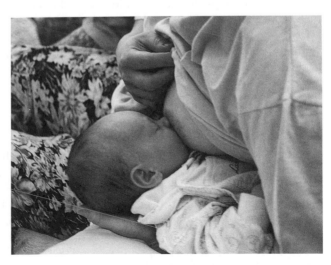

Often called the 'rugby ball' hold

The underarm position is useful when a toddler has to be attended to at the same time.

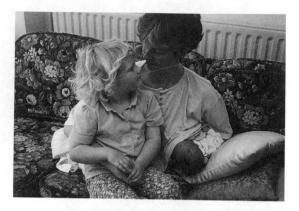

Baby in the underarm position

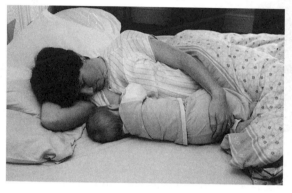

Feeding while lying down

With the mother lying on her side, the baby lies alongside and close to her. It is often useful to raise the breast from the mattress very slightly, by placing the short side of a pillow under the mother's ribs so that the edge of the pillow is at the junction of the breast and ribs. If the mother is lying on her left side, her right hand will be behind the baby's shoulders (so that his head can extend slightly) enabling her to direct the baby's chin to the lower breast. Again the nose is at the level of the nipple before the feed starts, so that as the baby opens his mouth the lower lip is well below the nipple.

Without moving the mother, the baby can feed from the upper breast, by raising his body with a cushion or pillow. For this position more active help from the midwife may be needed at first.

Breast support while feeding

Whether the mother will need to support her breast while feeding will depend on its size and shape. If support is needed she should be advised to:

- place her fingers flat on her rib cage at the base of the breast with her thumb uppermost, thus firming the inner tissue. She should take care not to move the breast towards the baby by exerting pressure with her thumb.

Occasionally it may be more helpful if she supports her breast with her hand from underneath and with the thumb above, ensuring that both are well behind the areola. She can then make the breast into a shape for the baby to latch on to, directing the nipple to the roof of the mouth.

Bringing the baby to the breast

- As the baby roots for the breast his lips or tongue should be allowed to touch the nipple and then be moved slightly away from it again, which will stimulate him to open his mouth wide.

- He is now brought back to the breast again with one quick but smooth movement, aiming his tongue and lower jaw as far as possible from the base of the nipple. His tongue will move over his lower lip to 'scoop up' the nipple and as much breast as possible. This will ensure that he has enough breast tissue in his mouth for his tongue to reach the lactiferous ducts within the breast.

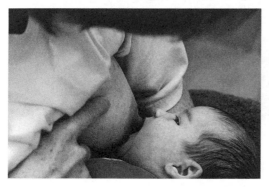

In the early days this manoeuvre may have to be repeated several times until good positioning is achieved, but at each attempt the baby's mouth must be moved away from the breast, so that the mouth opens wide again.

Gaping for the breast

The mother's recognition of correct positioning

- She feels a strong, (perhaps strange) and painless 'drawing' sensation as the baby scoops up the nipple and breast tissue, draws it into his mouth and begins to suckle.

- If there is any areola visible, she will see more above the top lip than below the bottom.

- The baby's nose hardly touches the breast.

- The chin is well in contact with the breast.

The cheeks remain full during suckling and the angle at the corner of the lips is wide (more than 100° degrees).

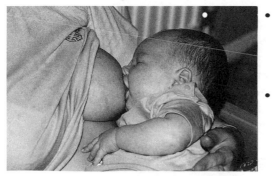

- The whole of the lower jaw moves - right up to the ears and occasionally even the ear lobe moves

- Swallowing *may* be heard but this only indicates that milk is flowing, not that the positioning is necessarily correct.

The well positioned baby

51

The midwife's recognition of correct positioning

In addition to all the above the midwife will also see that:

- More of the areola is visible above than below the baby's lips, if the mother has a large areola.

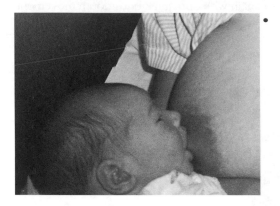

- She may see that the lower lip of the baby is curled outwards, but this is not always visible if the baby is close to the breast.

A well positioned baby whose mother has a large areola

Recognition of nipple sucking

In contrast, the baby who is nipple sucking may:

- continue to make little sucks, as if sucking a dummy

- not change the rhythm of his sucking

- purse his lips (The angle of the corner of the mouth will be less than 90° degrees)

- draw in his cheeks while sucking

- cause his mother pain

- manifest his frustration at not having his hunger satisfied by either becoming sleepy and ceasing to suck, or by coming off the breast and crying.

...and finally

Once the baby is correctly attached, the midwife should check that the mother is still relaxed, that her shoulders are not raised, that the weight if the baby is being supported on her thigh or the pillow and not taken by her arms which will tire, and that her calf muscles are not under tension (It might be useful to get her to take a couple of deep breaths, if she is tense). Muscular tension will not prevent the mother from breastfeeding but it makes the whole process more tiring than it need be.

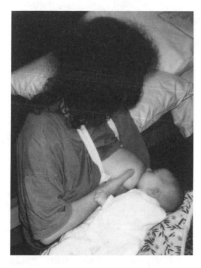

Mother supporting a heavy breast with a sling

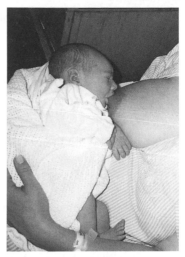

The baby has finished his feed and is coming off the breast

When she is feeding the baby comfortably, praise her (and her baby), admire her developing skills (if appropriate) and reinforce all the points that enabled her (or will enable her) to position the baby at the breast correctly herself.

Expressing breastmilk

While a mother is feeding a baby directly from the breast, learning to express breastmilk is a skill which may be useful for a variety of reasons. Dr Savage King suggests that all mothers should learn to express breastmilk.

(During my early days as a practising midwife, mothers were always taught to express colostrum by hand towards the end of their pregnancy to 'clear the ducts'. Once the baby was born they were given a small bowl after every feed to express any remaining milk in their breasts to encourage a good milk supply. This was in the days when feeding was restricted and expressing was designed to overcome the problems that might have resulted from this!)

Today, if a mother needs or wants to express breastmilk she is more likely to use one of a variety of hand or electric breast pumps available. However, hand expressing is a simple and cheap and convenient way to obtain breastmilk, without having to rely on gadgets, which may be unavailable, expensive, unreliable and which need to be sterilized after use.

Expressing breastmilk might be useful or necessary for a variety of reasons:

- the baby is unable to suckle directly from the breast i.e. because the baby is born prematurely or has an abnormality such as a cleft lip or palate and is unable to suck well

- the baby is sick and hospitalized and the mother cannot stay with the baby for 24 hours of the day

- to keep up the milk supply when the mother is sick, hospitalized or is temporarily separated from the baby

- to relieve engorgement

- to soften full breasts prior to a feed to aid correct positioning of the baby

- to relieve a blocked duct

- to rest the breasts, when the nipples have been traumatized and are too painful for direct breastfeeding

- to collect milk for someone else to give to the baby when the mother has planned to be away for an evening out

- to collect and store milk for the time when she is going back to work

- to collect milk for donation to a milk bank

Expressing breastmilk by hand

To help the mother understand how to express her milk, it is always useful to explain to her the basic anatomy and physiology of the breast and lactation. An understanding of how her breasts functions and how sensitive her body is to the needs of her baby helps to give her confidence in her ability to express and provide milk.

If the baby is unable to breastfeed at first she should be taught this skill as soon as possible and while the breasts are soft. An American nurse tells her mothers that the colostrum she expresses, even just the few drops are like 'liquid gold!'

Whether the need for expressed milk is an emergency, or for a planned reason, it helps to learn the skill of hand expressing when the breasts are soft, ideally, before the milk comes in or when they become soft again later.

Preparing to express milk

HELPING TO STIMULATE THE LET-DOWN REFLEX

Many mothers feel rather self-conscious about expressing milk and handling their breasts and need privacy to relax. Ideally one midwife, experienced in expressing, should show the mother how to use hands and watch her expressing some milk/ colostrum.

It may help to:

- apply a warm flannels to the breasts

- stroke the breast gently towards the nipple (Renfrew, 1990)

- massage the breasts gently with the three middle fingers in a circular motion from the edges of the breasts. Care must be taken to massage gently, so as not to cause friction and skin soreness

- briefly and gently role the nipple

- have the baby nearby, if he/she is already breastfeeding or just thinking about the baby acts on the neuro-hormonal reflex.

Rolling the fist gently over the breast towards the areola may stimulate the release of oxytocin, but care must be taken to avoid skin friction. Sandra Lang demonstrates this with the clenched fist at right angles to the chest and rolling it towards the nipple (Lang, personal communication).

Cleanliness

Although breastmilk contains many substances which combat infection, it is essential that *expressing the milk is as clean a process as possible*, particularly if it is to be stored for a period of time.

- The hands must be washed and dried on a clean towel

- The container for the milk should be sterilized.

At first a wide open bowl may be best. As the mother feels more confident, she may be able to direct the flow of milk directly into a wide mouthed bottle. The type of container depends on the milk flow, which may spurt up, down, sideways or forwards!

- hands must be washed and dried on a clean or paper towel

Renfrew suggests that the first attempts are made in a bath or under the shower, because warmth is relaxing (Renfrew, 1990). Later, sitting comfortably on a chair and leaning slightly forward, a cup should be held close to the breast. A towel placed beneath the breast will catch any drips.

To express milk

- the mother should search for the ampullae beneath the areola (They are not so easily palpable during the first couple of days, but once the milk comes in will feel 'knotty').

- the fingers of the other hand should cradle the breast from underneath with the forefinger at the lower edge of the areola and the thumb at the upper edge. The exact position depends on the size of the areola, the aim being to exert gentle pressure on to the inner edge of the ampullae.

At the same time Renfrew also suggests that the whole hand presses back and in towards the chest wall.

- With a steady rhythmic movement of pressure and release milk will start flowing. This unusual use of the fingers will tire them but they will gradually strengthen. Breaking the rhythm and massaging the breasts again, particularly where they feel firm (once the milk has come in) will give them a rest. As there are 15-20 lobes, there are 15-20 ampullae and the fingers and thumb may need to be rotated as the ampullae empty.

- Expressing should be pain free.

- Care should be taken that the fingers do not slip down on to the nipple and damage the narrowing ducts.

- In the first few days the mother may express only a few drops. As the skill is learned, the time it takes to express enough for a feed gets shorter. Just as with demand feeding no time can be set, but as the flow becomes slower she can switch to the other side.

- The frequency of expressing milk depends on the reason for expressing in the first place.

At the same time, she must remember that, the more milk she expresses the more milk she will make.

Like all skills, expressing takes practice and only a small minority of women are not able to express milk. Many mothers who say they are unable to express just need to be shown how to do it more effectively.

Collection and storage of expressed milk

Expressed milk should be stored in sterilized containers, preferably with an air tight lid. (Hard plastic containers with solid lids show the least loss of immunological factors during storage, reduce the risk of contamination and reduce the risk of exposure of the nutrients in the milk to oxidation (Garza, 1982; Goldblum, 1981). It should be clearly labelled with the date and time of collection, and the mother's name, and used in rotation.

Storing the milk in feeding sized portions will minimize the waste.

Although it is advisable to refrigerate expressed milk as soon as possible, unless it is to be used within the hour, researchers who have examined the effect of storage time and temperature on bacterial counts in human milk report that term human milk can be safely left at room temperature for 6-10 hours, and preterm milk for up to 4 hours (in the tropics) (Pittard, 1985; Larson. 1984; Barger and Bull, 1987; Ajusi, 1989; Nwankwo, 1988).

Once stored in the fridge it can safely remain there for 24-48 hours, after which is should be frozen if it is to be kept. Again, the studies which have examined the rate of growth of bacteria in refrigerated human milk found that it could, in fact, be left for much longer than is generally thought - up to five days (Berkow, 1984; Jensen and Jensen, 1992).

Frozen milk for preterm infants should be used within three months and within six months for term infants. Most home and hospital freezers are incapable of reaching - 20°C, the temperature below which milk enzymes cease to be active, in consequence milk fat continues to be hydrolysed even when frozen. The denatured fat may cause the milk to have a soapy flavour or even appear rancid when it is thawed.

The milk can be thawed when required by standing it in a jug of warm water. If the milk container is held under a running tap, care should be taken not to wet the lid, so that there is no risk of the water contaminating the milk when the lid is removed (Sigman, 1989; Quan, 1992; Nemethy and Clore, 1990). It should never be thawed in hot water nor in a microwave oven.

Once thawed, unused milk must be discarded. Milk, whether fresh or thawed, that has been in contact with the infant's saliva, must be discarded if unused during a feeding.

Adapted from: Recommendations for collection, storage and handling of a mother's milk for her own infant in the hospital setting. 1993 The Human milk Banking Association of North America Inc. PO Box 370464, West Hartford, CT 06137-0464.

CHAPTER TEN

Care Practices Which Influence Breastfeeding

Since the first publication in 1975 of the five-yearly Infant Feeding Surveys conducted by the Office of Population Censuses and Surveys (OPCS), it has been possible to examine the changes that have occurred in breastfeeding practices. At the same time the surveys have drawn attention to their effect on the length of breastfeeding (Martin, 1978, 1982 and 1988; White, 1992). The findings support the importance of self-regulated/demand feeding and rooming-in for the success of breastfeeding. They also highlight the adverse impact of other practices on the duration of breastfeeding, for example delays in starting breastfeeding after birth or giving complementary feeds. Yet even some recently published paediatric textbooks, in which breastfeeding guidelines are proposed, are not based on current research findings. Nevertheless, many hospitals do have breastfeeding guidelines which include good, research-based practices. Regrettably, only one in ten of these hospitals have also given in-service training to the staff to implement the guidelines, according to an unpublished survey of 193 Maternity Units undertaken by the Joint Breastfeeding Initiative in 1992. If staff do not understand the reasons for changes in practice or how to implement them, it is not surprising that guidelines are often ignored (Beeken, 1992).

I would like to suggest that the lack of knowledge of the total process of breastfeeding and its application to practice needs to be addressed by means of an intensive training programme for health professionals.

It is not uncommon, for example, to find that both midwives and mothers are under the misconception that the quantity of colostrum produced in the first two or three days is insufficient to sustain the baby. It is forgotten that the forces of evolution acting on mothers and their newborn babies have resulted in a finely balanced symbiotic relationship (Montagu, 1986). The mother's body nourishes and grows the baby in utero for nine months and then produces the food that is sufficient to sustain the baby. Throughout pregnancy the forces of evolution create a fine balance between mother and fetus, which continues after birth. Ashley Montagu describes this eloquently in his book *Touching - The Human Significance of Skin*:

> 'The biological unity, the symbiotic relationship, maintained by the mother and conceptus during pregnancy does not cease at birth, but becomes - indeed, is naturally designed to become - even more intensified and interoperative than during uterogestation....Her whole organism has been readied to minister to the

infant's needs....For the newborn, what better reassurance can there be than the support of the mother and the satisfaction of suckling at her breast, what better promise of good things to come?'

(He argues that at the birth the human baby has completed only half of it's gestation period but must be born, because it's head would otherwise not be able to negotiate the birth canal.)

With few exceptions a mother's body produces sufficient colostrum to match the baby's needs, with an average volume of 7mls per feed on the first day (Houston, 1983). Even though this may appear to be very little, it matches the size of the baby's stomach which has the dimension of his fist.

Unfortunately, the extensive use of formula feeds has resulted in midwives seeing much larger volumes of milk taken at each feed on the first day of an artificially fed baby's life. They may subsequently find it difficult to believe that the (physiologically small) volume of colostrum that the mother provides at each feed is 'enough'.

It may be the case that once the stomach (which is a distensible organ) has been expanded, the baby may not be satisfied unless it is distended again at the next feed. If this is so, it is yet another argument against the use of top-up feeds of formula for breastfed babies.

Frequency of feeding

The normal healthy baby has a strong instinct for survival. It is expressed by a loud vocal demand for food as the blood sugar falls (not all crying is indicative of hunger, the baby may also be communicating that he is in discomfort or lonely). In the past mothers have been instructed to ignore the cry for food by those who thought a baby should be 'trained', or that feeding should be 'organized'.

Since the end of the eighteenth century feeding patterns have changed from demand to strict feeding schedules and back again (Fildes, 1986). Between the 1920s and 1970s rigid feeding schedules dominated hospital practices, although demand feeding practices did exist. For example, in 1956 Professor R Illingworth wrote: 'We cannot see any point in leaving a baby howling for food because the alarm clock has not said that it is time for him to feel hungry'.

In the 1950s I had the good fortune to work with a midwife, Olive Rogers, who taught me that babies have the ability to regulate their own feeding patterns. Since then I have had many opportunities in the private and public sector to observe this for myself and teach others this fundamental truth.

Babies show great variation in the frequency of their feeds during the first 48 hours, ranging from 0 - 11 feeds/24 hours (Modal 4.3. ± 2.5) on the first day and 1 - 22 feeds/24 hours (Modal 7.4 ± 2.5) on the second day (Yamauchi, 1990). There is some evidence that frequent early feeding is of benefit. Neonatal jaundice and weight loss are less likely (Salaryia, 1978) and the total duration of breastfeeding may be increased (White et al, 1992).

Once feeding is established, at between four and six weeks, many babies settle into a fairly regular pattern of feeding. This may vary considerably between babies from three, four or even five hourly feeds.

In the early evening it is not unusual for the interval between feeds to be shorter than the rest of the day.

In Great Britain a change to demand or self-regulated feeding is being adopted only slowly. National surveys undertaken by the Office of Population Censuses and Surveys have found an increase from 68 per cent in 1980 to 90 per cent in 1990. Mothers have reacted favourably to these flexible feeding systems and this change may be one of the reasons why fewer mothers abandon breastfeeding during the first six weeks, 52 per cent in 1975 and 25 per cent in 1990 (White, 1992).

Duration of a feed

In the first few weeks of lactation, many mothers have a surplus of milk and babies are often satisfied with the milk obtained from one breast. The length of the feed varies considerably from one mother-infant pair to another and depends on the rate of milk release by the mother and the rate of milk demand by the baby (Woolridge, 1982).

When using a demand or self-regulating feeding regime therefore, the length of feeds varies not only from one feed to the next but from one baby to another. The baby who has been well attached will let go of the first breast when he has had enough from that side. His body language will let the mother know whether he is satisfied – if he cries or searches for more milk, the second side should be offered. It can take up to six weeks for the breasts to reach the stage of having 'learned' how much milk to produce for the needs of the individual baby and to establish a pattern of feeding. There is, however, no hard and fast rule. (Some mothers can find the uncertainty of not knowing when the baby wants to feed difficult to cope with. In this case she should not be prevented from trying to feed her baby on a fixed feeding schedule, knowing that she has the freedom to make adjustments as necessary.)

A baby who stays at the breast for prolonged periods without coming off spontaneously or a baby who wants to feed very frequently through the day and night, is probably not positioned correctly. He may therefore only obtain some foremilk, which does not sustain him for very long and drives him to feed frequently. Apart from anything else, it is likely to make his mother very tired. The OPCS survey 'Infant Feeding 1990' found that from the second week onwards, mothers reported 'excessive tiredness' to be one of the most common reasons for discontinuing breastfeeding (White et al, 1992).

However, incorrect positioning and the subsequent need for frequent feeds (of low fat foremilk) may cause other problems.

Frequent, poorly positioned feeds may cause nipple damage, will not use the breast efficiently and may give rise to engorgement and/or mastitis.

As a result the baby may not be able to consume enough calories and may eventually cease to gain or even lose weight. The large volumes of milk that the baby consumes in an effort to obtain the calories he needs may give rise to vomiting, abdominal discomfort ('wind'), and frequent, explosive stools (Woolridge and Fisher, 1988).

Rooming-in

The concept of keeping mother and baby together continuously on a postnatal ward has also been demonstrated to have beneficial effects on mother-infant interaction and breastfeeding (Klaus et al, 1972; De Chateau, 1977; Keefe, 1987). Rooming-in had been advocated by Dr Spock in 1951. However, he felt it to be difficult to establish as it would involve many changes in hospital administration and philosophy. He also considered a long planning and testing period to be necessary.

It has to be said that rooming-in as a concept of care was introduced in a haphazard way in Britain. It has increased from 17 per cent in 1980 to 63 per cent in 1990 but has not kept pace with the increase in the number of units in which demand feeding was the policy, 90 per cent in 1990. It is therefore not surprising that the 1990 OPCS survey also found 45 per cent of breastfed babies had been given a formula feed (White, 1992).

Separating mothers from their babies for part or most of the time is likely to contribute to this practice and will shorten the duration of breastfeeding (White, 1992; Begley, 1993; De Chateau, 1977).

The *advantages* of rooming-in, keeping mother and baby together continuously, are well documented. She learns about her baby's needs and how to care for him, being close she sees and knows that he is alright and can touch or pick him up for a cuddle.

As early as 1972 Klaus et al. published a study which showed the beneficial effect of rooming-in on mother-baby interaction, (Klaus, 1972; Klaus and Kennell, 1982), while a Swedish study found mothers to be more confident and caring (Waldenstrom, 1991).

Extended contact – in contrast to the earlier custom of keeping babies in a nursery between feeds – can also increase an interest in breastfeeding (Procianoy, 1983; Elander, 1984).

Rooming-in can be said to be the pre-requisite for demand feeding. It is clearly easier for the mother to feed her baby whenever he shows signs of hunger when the baby's cot is next to her bed.

Rooming-in and night feeds

It is still not uncommon for breastfed babies to be removed to the nursery at night and given a formula feed if they wake while their mother is asleep. This may be one of the reasons why so many breastfed babies (45 per cent) were reported to have been given a formula feed whilst in hospital (White, 1992). Even though this may be done for the best of motives (i.e. to let the mother sleep) it is clear that this practice shortens the duration of breastfeeding (De Chateau, 1977; White, 1992; Begley, 1993).

Ball (1987) found that mothers who suffered from sleep deprivation were described by midwives as being unduly distressed about feeding their baby. The resulting exhaustion raised their anxiety levels and reduced their ability to learn. Under these circumstances, it is only too common for mothers to be overwhelmed by breastfeeding problems and resorting to formula feeding becomes a real temptation.

This situation could be prevented if the policy of rooming-in was implemented intelligently.

If the mother is tired or even exhausted from the birth, all she should have to do is breastfeed the baby. If the mother wishes, the carer can pick up, change and settle the baby, until the mother is ready to do these tasks herself.

The 'That's Life' survey (Boyd and Sellers, 1982) collected the opinion of 6000 self selected mothers and found that many women did not want the baby to be beside them at night but particularly liked the arrangement where the baby stayed in the nursery and was brought to them to feed.

Advantages of night feeds

Most mothers accept that night feeds are an integral part of having a new baby. It takes a while for babies to learn the difference between night and day and in the early weeks about half of the 24 hour milk-requirement has to be met by night feeds.

Because attitudes of mind affect feelings it may be useful for a mother to know that night feeds have some advantages for her as well:

- more frequent 'emptying' of the breast reduces engorgement when the milk first comes in (Lawrence, 1994)

- breastfeeding has a soporific effect on the mother and the quality of sleep improves. This may be explained by the release of dopamine which is said to be involved in the mechanism of oxytocin release (Corsini, 1977; Bourne, 1982)

- prolactin levels are higher at night and ensure good milk production (Howie, 1982)

- exclusive breastfeeding raises prolactin levels which in turn suppresses luteinizing hormone release, thus preventing ovulation (Howie, 1982).

Bedding-in

Hugh Jolly, formerly Consultant Paediatrician at the Charing Cross Hospital, encouraged mothers to have their baby in bed with them, a rare practice in this country's maternity units but common in the Far East. Dr Jolly also encouraged the family bed for the baby:

> 'Psychoanalysts may be firm in their advice that parents must never allow their children into their beds, but those who have practised it know better and have not had any dire consequences to face - just the opposite.'

However, if after birth the mother is exhausted or if she had Pethidine towards the end of labour this practice is contra-indicated for obvious reasons.

This also applies if night sedation is given, as she may sleep heavily and not be aware of the baby next to her. Nor should the baby share the parents' bed if they sleep on a water mattress, have consumed large amounts of alcohol or if the baby is immobilized in plaster.

If the parents have decided to share their bed with the baby from the beginning of the night, they should be warned that once the baby is used to being close to them at night, it may take two, three or even four years, before the child is ready to sleep in a bed on his own. Abruptly changing the child's sleeping habits, insisting that he go to sleep in his own bed earlier than he is ready, would cause considerable distress.

On the other hand, parents who simply take the baby into their bed if he wakes after they have gone to sleep, will not be sharing their bed for the first part of the night and will cease to share it at all when the baby stops waking for night feeds.

CHAPTER ELEVEN

Recognition of the Healthy Baby

A word-picture of a healthy baby
- He is alert with a good colour and a silky skin.
- His trunk and limbs are covered with a layer of firm fat. Efficient muscles are revealed by his active movements.
- His skin is warm and he breathes easily.
- The skin of his skull is firm.
- His abdomen is prominent but soft.
- He passes urine and stool without discomfort.
- He sleeps well, wakes, eats, is satisfied, lies awake for a while and sleeps again.
- He cries at intervals for hunger, loneliness, discomfort, or more obscure reasons, but not for long and not for more than one or two hours in the 24 hours.
- This good to look at, happy, lively baby, eats with appetite and is gaining weight.

(From Wood, C.B.S., Walker-Smith, J.A. (1981). *MacKeith's Infant Feeding and Feeding Difficulties.*)

The growth of the baby
Weight gain and loss
Until birth all the nutrients essential for growth are transmitted to the fetus intravenously via the placenta which also returns the waste products into the maternal circulation. From the moment of birth, the baby's body has undergone enormous (internal) change and from the first feed of colostrum, the baby also has to cope with digestion.

Normal healthy babies, weighing between 3000 -4000 grams may to lose five to ten per cent of their birth weight in the first three to four days.

This is said to be due to:

- the passage of meconium

- loss of water, possibly as a result of changes in volume and distribution of water in the body (Shaffer, 1987)

- feeding practices and the amount of colostrum the baby takes (Maisels, 1985).

It has also been that the degree of weight loss correlates directly with the timing of the first breastfeed (Enzunga, 1990). In other words, the sooner the baby has his first breastfeed, the less weight he loses. Furthermore, unrestricted breastfeeding has been shown to increase early milk production and promotes infant weight gain by comparison with a restrictive feeding schedule (de Carvalho, 1983).

As the milk comes in the baby begins to grow by an average of 20 - 30 grams a day. Many babies have doubled their birthweight by about four months. However all babies vary and some may grow more slowly.

Some caution needs to be used in interpreting the weight gain of a breastfed baby when plotted on standard growth charts. The weight and height criteria most commonly used in the United Kingdom are the Tanner standards. These were collected between 1952 and 1954 on only 80 boys and 80 girls and the measurements were made only at three month intervals. Tanner himself did not consider such data as suitable for interpreting the finer details of growth in very young babies, and certainly not as a yardstick for judging the adequacy of breastfeeding (Whitehead and Paul, 1984).

The DARLING study (Dewey, 1992) compared two matched groups of infants who were either breastfed or formula fed during the first 12 months of their lives. Neither group were given solids before four months. The groups had similar weight gains during the first three months but breastfed infants gained less rapidly during the remainder of the first year. Length gain was similar between groups thus weight for length scores suggested that breastfed infants were leaner. This study adds to the growing evidence (from the US, Canada, Australia, Finland, Sweden and the UK) that charts compiled using data from a time when formula feeding and the early introduction of solids were common are inappropriate for assessing the growth of breastfed infants.

The weight loss of newborn babies was studied in a teaching hospital in Zaire (Avoa, 1990). The effect of giving four simple breastfeeding instructions to a group of mothers of 162 children was compared with a group of mothers with 142 children who did not get special instructions. The educational intervention was provided to mothers in the hospital on alternate weeks only. It required one to two minutes and was given during the immediate perinatal period, usually in the delivery room. There were no other differences in the care given to the two groups.

The instructions, given to the mother by a midwife or senior student were:

- breastfeeding provides an ideal nutrition

- drinking colostrum is beneficial to the health of the baby

- suckling stimulates the production of breastmilk

- the baby should be nursed as soon after delivery as conveniently possible and frequently thereafter.

The study found:

- the babies in the intervention group lost 3.8 per cent of their birth weight before beginning to gain weight.

- the babies whose mother did not receive the instructions lost 6.2 per cent of their birth weight.

CHAPTER TWELVE

Helping a Mother to Overcome Breastfeeding Problems

The issues

Becoming a mother is a major life event which will totally transform the pattern of a woman's life (Holmes, 1967).

In her book, *Reactions to Motherhood*, Ball (1987) quotes the reactions and feelings of one 23 year old first-time mother:

> 'Being a mother is harder work than I had imagined it to be. I now realize that a baby definitely is not a doll to be paraded round in fancy frills! At times the baby is a real handful and when my husband goes to work after a rough night I feel depressed and unable to cope...But when the baby is awake and looking at me, or asleep in my arms, I get a feeling of utter peace and contentment and realize he is worth it after all'.

In the early days following birth the mother's body undergoes tremendous physical and hormonal changes (Pitt, 1978). At the same time the mother must learn to care for her newborn baby, whose only means of communication is body language and crying. Schools rarely include this aspect of parenthood in their curriculum and little, if anything, may be taught about baby care in parent craft classes.

The mother has to come to terms emotionally with the birth, which may have left her in a state of elation or disappointment. Sometimes the combination of a sore perineum, possible difficulties with sitting and walking, coupled with the realization of the responsibility which will be hers for many years to come can bring a fearful sense of anti-climax (Pitt, 1978). Breastfeeding adds yet another highly emotional aspect to this complex situation.

Yet postnatal care has been called the Cinderella of midwifery. For the midwife it is not an exciting period like labour. Today, the hospital midwife may not find much job satisfaction from working on a postnatal ward. Mothers are discharged within hours or one or two days unless they or their baby suffers from a complication. If the mother is not known to her from the antenatal period, it is not easy to have a genuine interest in her progress and the outcome of breastfeeding.

Postnatal care is truly very different from the so called Lying-in period of the past. Yet mothers have not changed. They still need an environment where self-confidence can grow while beginning to learn about their baby and acquire the new skills they need.

The individual care they receive and the help they are given in these early hours or days make a vital contribution to breastfeeding success. Rajan (1993) found that satisfaction with all aspects of midwifery care while in hospital to be an important factor in breastfeeding success - and its absence a significant contributor to failure. In this study of 1049 women, what they said they most needed was:

- clearer information
- non-conflicting advice
- correct practical support.

The above study supports the findings of the 'Infant Feeding 1985' (Martin and White, 1988) which found that many women stopped breastfeeding earlier than they would have liked as a result of problems that could have been prevented.

Assessment of the breastfeeding situation

To provide appropriate care for a breastfeeding woman, some knowledge of the mother's and baby's background may be useful (this could be obtained either from her care plan or by gentle questioning).

For instance:

- Is this her first baby?

- If not, did she breastfeed before?

- If so, when and why did she stop?

- Did she have a normal labour?

- What analgesia was given and when?

- What type of delivery did she have?

- Did the baby have problem at birth?

- When was the baby first put to the breast?

- Have there been any problems before the present time?

- What advice has already been given?

Listening to the mother with this background knowledge in mind makes it easier to get a more complete picture of her needs.

On the basis of her research, Rajan (1993) suggests that the women who are likely to need extra support and encouragement are those who have:

- experienced a difficult birth

- received pethidine during labour, particularly if this was within one hour of birth

- been separated from their baby for any reason.

Preventing problems

During the short time a woman stays in hospital, efforts should be made to devote at least 45 minutes of 'quality time' to teach her the basic physiology, practice and ground rules of breastfeeding. A leaflet with this information may help her to recall the information:

- a mother makes all the colostrum her baby needs. The size of the baby's stomach is roughly the size of his fist and matches the supply.

- colostrum not only provides the nutritional needs of the baby but gives him his first immunization against infection.

- the let-down reflex takes a few second to come into operation at first, but eventually just thinking about feeding will cause the milk to flow.

- if he is positioned properly he will take all the colostrum he needs and come off the breast spontaneously. After bringing up some wind, he may take the second side.

- the more often the baby is fed, the sooner the milk will come in and the more milk is produced. Conversely the less the baby feeds the less milk will be made.

The problem of time and shortage of staff is often cited as a reason for being unable to give help. However, time is generally found when the mother *has* problems. Could this time not be found earlier? How much better to prevent problems, as well as the ensuing stress, by giving breastfeeding a flying start!

General approach to breastfeeding problems

Before exploring a problem, the mother should be put at ease. Giving time may be a specially important factor, if the mother, and perhaps the baby, are distressed.

A crying baby should be calmed down. This is easier for the midwife to achieve than the mother. However, as this could undermine the mother's self-confidence, the midwife should explain that the baby recognizes her from the scent of her milk, which frustrates him if he hungry and cannot start feeding immediately. The midwife on the other hand does not smell of milk, making it easier to stop him crying.

Diverting the mother's attention at this stage also helps to relax her a little, if the situation has been fraught. Some aspect of the baby could be admired - the dimple in his cheeks, the curve of his eyelids or his lovely skin. Another way of diffusing some of the tension and anxiety is to inject a little humour into the situation, perhaps smiling at the funny faces the baby makes or his eagerness to find something to suck.

While giving the mother time to talk through her problem, the midwife can respond by repeating or reflecting some of the points the mother makes to:

i)   show the mother she is listening
ii)   check that she is correctly interpreting what the mother is saying.

It can also be helpful to find out what the mother's expectations were. Questions posed to explore the problem further should be open-ended – how, what and when. During the discussion criticism should be avoided, and whenever appropriate, a positive comment should be interjected (Hunter, 1994). All the while the midwife can keep one eye on the baby's behaviour and observe his well-being by his colour, muscle tone and respiration.

In order to help the mother, the midwife will need to know the following but the mother may have already given her much of this information already.

•   how often does the baby feed?

•   for how long does he feed?

•   does *he* terminate the feed?

•   does he feed from one or both breast?

•   does he prefer one side to the other?

•   how does it feel to feed him?

•   what advice has been given already, if any?

More specific questions can now be added, if necessary, depending on the problem, but the midwife should try to avoid bombarding the mother with too many questions.

It may become evident during the discussion that the mother actually knows what she wants to do to resolve the situation and just wants 'permission' to do so. Alternatively she could be asked a direct question: 'how do *you* think this problem could be solved?'. With patience, an answer may well be forthcoming and the suggestion worth trying. In my experience, most mothers have an inside knowledge they don't know exists!

Their need is an acknowledgement of their correct instinct for the needs of the baby. It will raise both their self-esteem and self-confidence in their mothering skill. The origin of conflicting advice often lies in offering advice too readily. If it is not what the mother wants to hear or if she somehow recognizes it to be incorrect, she will continue to ask the same question of another person, until she hears what she wants to hear.

'Information and support should go hand in hand; information being provided in the context of a helping relationship, which is characterized by respect, genuineness and empathy.' (Hunter 1994)

CHAPTER THIRTEEN

Milk Supply

Milk production

The volume of colostrum taken by the baby in the first 24 hours is approximately 7.5mls per feed (Houston, 1983). This increases to an average of 14mls, 38mls, 58mls and 70mls per feed over each of the following 24 hour periods (up to the fifth day), although the actual volume and the rate of increase may depend on the frequency of feeding and the efficiency of breast 'emptying' (Salaryia, 1978; Yamauchi and Yamaouchi, 1990). Only a very few mothers (between one and five per cent) do not develop sufficient glandular tissue for adequate milk production (Neifert, 1986).

Regulation of milk supply

Provided that there is no interference with the physiological process on which milk synthesis depends i.e. the baby has unrestricted access to and is correctly attached at the breast, initial milk production can be regulated both upwards and downwards as it adjusts to demand. Thus a woman with three babies to feed can produce three times as much milk in 24 hours as a woman with only one baby to feed (Saint, 1986).

Two separate mechanisms seem to be involved, *prolactin secretion* and *milk removal.*

Prolactin secretion

The level of prolactin in the mother's body has been rising throughout pregnancy and is at its peak at term. As the placental hormones leave the maternal circulation, milk production begins even if the baby does not go to the breast. However if the breasts are not used, the prolactin levels start to fall at the end of the first week and have returned to normal levels within two to three weeks postpartum (Lawrence, 1994).

Suckling, on the other hand, causes a surge in prolactin levels in the maternal blood stream, which slowly return to base-line levels over the next two hours (Howie, 1980). The more often the baby suckles, the more prolactin is released. However, although the presence of prolactin is essential for milk production, (bromocriptine, which abolishes prolactin secretion, will suppress lactation with 24-48 hours [Willmott, 1977]) there does not appear to be a precise, quantitative relationship between prolactin levels and milk volume (Howie, 1980b).

The prolactin response to suckling appears to be more marked in relation to feeds occurring after midday, which may explain the importance of night feeds in the maintenance of lactational amenorrhoea, but it is not correlated with milk volume during the day (Glasier, 1984). Moreover, as lactation progresses, both the prolactin response to suckling and the base-line levels diminish, although milk production continues unabated (Leake, 1983; Glasier, 1984).

Furthermore, an entirely satisfactory milk production has been found in women who initiated and maintained their lactation using a breastpump which failed to provide a prolactin discharge (Howie, 1980b).

Milk removal

In 1970 Applebaum wrote 'Drainage and not milk production is the sine qua non of successful breastfeeding'. A year later, Linzell and Peaker (1971) proposed that this was due to the presence of a local, autocrine inhibitor in the milk (of goats). If this was allowed to build up, milk synthesis was reduced. Subsequent research has strongly supported an endocrine model for the short term control of milk synthesis in women (Wilde et al., 1988; Prentice et al., 1989; Daly et al., 1993).

The development of a rapid computerized breast measurement system, which measures the changes in breast volume between breastfeeds, has made it possible to measure milk synthesis in the mother as distinct from consumption in the infant (by test weighing) (Arthur et al.,1989).

It has subsequently been established that the rates of milk synthesis vary markedly between breasts, vary markedly between inter-feed intervals and are positively related to the degree to which the breast is emptied.

Furthermore, a mother's breast can and does produce more milk than the infant usually requires. Drewett and Woolridge (1981) found that no matter which breast the infant had first, all the babies in their study took less from the second breast than from the first (as determined by test-weighing). In all seven of the mothers studied by Daly et al (1993) at least one of their breasts contained significant volumes of milk available to the infant after almost every feed. Both these studies demonstrate that the amount of milk consumed was not regulated by the amount of milk available but by the baby himself.

The mean rate of milk synthesis for an individual breast was, on average for all mothers, 64 per cent of the maximum rate of synthesis observed for that breast during that 24 hour study.

Thus milk production could be readily increased to accommodate an increase in the demand for milk by the infant, and in a much shorter time period than had previously been supposed (i.e. hours rather than days). The more milk the baby removed at a feed, the greater the degree of milk synthesis after the feed.

Over production

True over-production of milk is rare but an over-supply may be created by faulty feeding practices, such as taking the baby off the first breast before he stops feeding spontaneously and then offering the second breast.

Not only is the mother likely to experience considerable discomfort but because milk production and milk removal are out of step she may develop mastitis as back pressure on the ductal system causes milk to seep out of the ducts and into the connective tissue, causing an inflammatory reaction.

Additionally, this pattern of feeding may result in an unhappy baby. If the baby is taken off the first breast before he has finished, he will not have reached the higher fat hind milk that comes at the end of the feed, but mainly low-fat foremilk, which has a rapid transit through the stomach and duodenum (Woolridge and Fisher, 1988).

He will then have to take, or try and take, a much larger volume of milk from the second breast than he might otherwise have done in order to obtain the calories he needs. In consequence he will have consumed a much larger quantity of lactose per feed than he 'intended', as the concentration of lactose does not change during the course of a feed. The excess lactose may be fermented by bacteria in the gut, causing 'colic', wind and explosive (sometimes green) stools. The baby may respond to this pattern of feeding by:

- wanting to feed frequently, as the foremilk contains little fat to sustain him

- being generally unhappy and crying, drawing up his legs in apparent pain with colic

- having frequent and loose stools (not diarrhoea, when the stools are watery)

- bringing up milk during winding and at the end of the feed (because he cannot contain the volume he has taken in order to try and obtain the calories)

- either gaining weight rapidly or failing to gain weight.

The solution lies in allowing the baby to finish the first breast first, and come off the breast spontaneously, before offering the second, so that he receives a balanced feed. Starting each feed on alternate breasts at consecutive feeds reduces the over-stimulation of the breasts and solves the problem physiologically.

Too little milk

Milk insufficiency is the most common reason for giving up breastfeeding from the first week to the end of the ninth month (Martin, 1992). 30 per cent of the mothers gave this as the reason for the first two days in the 1990 OPCS survey. Surprisingly this increased to 47 per cent during the next four days, the days when the breasts feel full with the influx of milk. During the next two months the rise continues and reaches a peak of 74 per cent.

Not only do these figures reflect the general lack of confidence mothers have in their ability to provide sufficient milk for their baby, but also the lack of support which might have overcome this problem. On-going studies in rural Gambia (Prentice, 1988) have found that even chronically undernourished mothers are able to produce sufficient milk for their baby. Although the mean birth weight of babies born to under-nourished mothers is lower compared to babies born in Cambridge, the growth curve of breastfed babies is parallel for the first two months following birth.

Woolridge (1993) has often observed that 'insufficient milk' was the main reason why mothers came to his breastfeeding problem clinic. In most cases he found this to be due to incorrect feeding practices (personal communication).

It may also be the case that mothers give 'not having enough milk' as their reason for ceasing to breastfeed, when in fact there was some other reason, because they know that this will be regarded sympathetically.

At the same time the midwife must be aware that occasionally she may be caring for one of the very few women who really cannot produce sufficient milk for her baby (Neifert, 1986).

Insufficient milk

During the two or three days after the birth, it is difficult for a new mother to believe that her breasts produce sufficient nourishment for her baby. Her breasts are soft and unchanged and colostrum is unlikely to leak. This applies particularly when she sees the amount of milk a bottle fed baby takes from the first day.

Generally, it is the mother's interpretation of the baby's behaviour, that leads her to think that she does not have enough milk/colostrum.

She may complain that the baby:

* cries a lot

* wants to feed all the time

* takes too long over a feed

* quickly falls asleep at the breast

* soon cries again when he comes off the breast

* takes a formula feed eagerly, if offered and settles.

The adequacy of colostrum intake cannot be determined by criteria that assess fluid intake. The baby will pass very little urine as circulating levels of anti-diuretic hormone are high after birth. However colostrum may well stimulate the baby's gut to pass meconium if this was not passed at birth.

At this stage the midwife needs to know whether:

- breastfeeding hurts

- the baby's behaviour at the breast suggests that he is well attached

- the baby leaves the breast spontaneously.

After the first day she might ask whether:

- the colour of the meconium is beginning to change from black to green, then brown and by the fourth day to yellow

- the baby has wet nappies and how often they have to be changed

- the colour of the urine is pale or concentrated.

The above observations take only a short time. But the attention and concern of the midwife will already help to calm the situation. To make the correct assessment of the situation *the midwife also needs to observe a feed* to:

i)   assess why the mother finds it difficult to position the baby and help her learn this skill to ensure an adequate *milk transfer from mother to baby*.

ii)   to explain to her again the main points which lead to successful breastfeeding (see Chapter 9).

Later stages of lactation

In the normal progression of lactation the following changes are normal:

- the duration of the feeds may become much shorter, as the feeding technique becomes more efficient

- the frequency of feeds subsides

- the marked contrast in the breasts between 'about to feed' and 'just fed' diminishes and the breasts are softer for more of the time

- the breasts may become smaller

- the mother loses some of the weight she has put on in pregnancy.

Test-weighing

Test weighing the baby before and after the feed, to assess whether the baby is taking too little or too much, used to be a common practice but is no longer considered useful for three main reasons (Inch and Renfrew, 1989):

i)   it is likely to be inaccurate over a 24 hour period unless electronic scales are used (Houston et al., 1983; Whitfield al., 1981).

ii)   the actual energy requirements for an individual baby may be difficult to assess and investigations suggest that they have been over-estimated (Whitehead, 1981; Butte, 1984).

iii)   supplementary feeding is more likely to be introduced reducing the milk supply still further with the greater likelihood that the mother will give up breastfeeding (De Chateau, 1977; White, 1990).

Complementary and supplementary feeding

Complementary feed - giving the baby a formula feed immediately after a breastfeed.

Supplementary feed - giving the baby a formula feed in place of a breastfeed

Giving artificial feeds to breastfed babies has been a common custom for very many years. Illingworth (1954) deplored this practice and considered it should be exceptional particularly in the first five days. He wrote:

> 'If the baby is satisfied with a good feed of cow's milk, he will suck less well at the breast and the breast will then be less well emptied'.

Since then several studies have demonstrated that breastfeeding women whose babies are given complementary bottle feeds are likely to stop breastfeeding sooner than those whose babies are exclusively breastfed (Sloper, 1977; West, 1980; Begley, 1993; Blomquist, 1994).

The OPCS Infant Surveys (Martin, 1982, 1988; White, 1992) also found a strong association between the giving of bottles and mothers who stopped breastfeeding in the first two weeks following birth.

In spite of this, 45 per cent of breastfed babies born in British hospitals were given bottle feeds (White, 1992).

Giving additional fluids to a breastfed baby does nothing to solve breastfeeding problems, it is likely to make them worse.

The *mother* may be given the impression that either

i)   her milk supply is insufficient

ii)   the quality is not good enough and subsequently if baby cries at the breast he 'obviously' prefers the bottle.

The *mother's breasts* are more likely to become overfull or even engorged, which will make attachment more difficult, and ultimately milk production will be reduced if milk removal does not keep pace with production.

If the *baby* has been continually frustrated in his attempts to obtain nourishment from the breast due to poor positioning, or has had other unpleasant experiences at the breast (such as force applied to the baby's head when fixing, or obstruction of breathing as a result of head flexion), and is then offered a bottle, he may then demonstrate his preference for the less traumatic bottlefeed by refusing the breast (Woolridge, 1993).

CHAPTER FOURTEEN

Painful Breastfeeding

It is not uncommon for the enjoyment of breastfeeding to be marred by transient pain and *tenderness of the nipples* (Gunther, 1945; Illingworth, 1956).

Drewett et al (1988) found that *nipple pain* peaked at two days. But although it declined steadily to the fifteenth day, 20-25 per cent of women still had nipple pain on the fifteenth to thirtieth day (The causes of this pain were not investigated).

Breast discomfort when the milk comes in is generally associated with unresolved early feeding difficulties culminating in stasis due to poor milk transfer. Any stasis, whether during early or later lactation, can develop into *mastitis* (Thomsen, 1984). Finally, a *breast abscess* can develop in a minority of women.

The 'Infant Feeding 1990' survey (White, 1992) found the combination of sore nipples and painful breasts to be the second most common reason (30 per cent) for stopping breastfeeding in the first two weeks. An infection with Candida Albicans can also be source of pain in breasts and nipples.

Prevention of the breasts and nipple trauma

A well supporting bra may add to the mother's comfort, particularly once the milk comes in or if the breasts are large. It is important that no part of the bra 'digs into' the breast tissue. Bras with 'windows' have this tendency, which can lead to the obstruction of milk flow from one lobe with the consequences described below.

Keeping the nipple skin supple and healthy requires no special skill. Attempting to keep the nipple clean, by the use of soap and water or alcohol in some form, has been shown to increase, rather than decrease, the incidence of soreness (Newton, 1952). All the lotions, creams and sprays on the market have either not been evaluated or have been shown to be either useless or harmful (Inch, 1990). Using a little expressed milk on the nipple after a feed has been evaluated and shown to be of no benefit (Hewat and Ellis, 1987).

The following are best avoided:

a)   soap to clean the nipples because it tends to dry the skin and encourages it to crack.

b)   plastic-backed breast pads as they keep the nipple moist and may encourage bacteria

c)   taking the baby off the breast, without first carefully breaking the suction

d)   the use of nipple shields which can further irritate an already sore nipple and are of no value whatsoever before the milk begins to flow.

Breast pain at the onset of feeding

A few mothers feel acute pain as the baby begins to suckle. The pain diminishes as soon as the let-down reflex comes into operation. It may be that the negative pressure exerted on the ducts before the milk flows is the cause of this pain (Woolridge, 1986). Getting the colostrum to flow by a little breast massage and expressing some drops of colostrum to encourage the let-down reflex, may reduce both the severity and duration of the pain. With rare exceptions, this situation resolves spontaneously within a few days.

Woolridge (1986) suggests that it may be corrected by 'improving positioning or degree of attachment on the breast so that the baby has a greater amount of tissue in his mouth from which to withdraw the milk more effectively'.

Sore/cracked nipples

These conditions are age-old problems. Fildes (1986) cites numerous sources which describe the nipple traumas women suffered in the sixteenth and seventeenth century. For example, nipple soreness, cracks and fissures, ulcers and loss of nipples and nipples obstructed or deformed by scar tissue from suckling a previous child.

Common misconceptions and assumptions regarding nipple trauma

Fair skin colouring and red/fair hair is often considered to predispose to sore nipples. Of 500 midwives attending refresher courses in 1990/1991, 37.4 per cent believed this to be true .

Yet the only studies which have investigated this belief have found no such association (Inch, 1989).

Restricting the duration of breast feeds, particularly in the first few days, has been an edict in the clinical situation and in textbooks on feeding from the beginning of this century (Fisher, 1993).

For generations, student midwives have been indoctrinated in this practice. Myles, in her *Textbook for Midwives*, (from 1st edition 1953 - 8th edition, 1975) admonished:

'Do not allow the baby to suck for longer than three minutes every six hours during the first two days. From the third day the infant should feed from both breasts not longer than ten minutes at each; longer than that will blister the nipples' (Myles, 1961).

Yet at the same time, (1956), R. and A. Illingworth, who admittedly were well ahead of their time on breastfeeding guidance and were early advocates of demand feeding, were writing about primitive tribes 'in which babies are allowed to suck as much as they like from birth onwards, there is no trouble from sore nipples'. Nevertheless, in their unit, the practice of restricting sucking time at the breast for the first three days was imposed by the 'nursing staff', who were afraid that otherwise mothers would develop sore nipples (Illingworth and Stone, 1952).

Gradually more liberal feeding practices have been introduced in UK hospitals, although even in 1990 10 per cent of hospitals were still using set feeding schedules (White, 1992).

The cause of sore/cracked nipples

Woolridge (1986b) clearly puts the responsibility for the development of nipple damage on frictional trauma as a result of incorrect attachment. The friction arises when the baby has been unable to obtain sufficient breast tissue to form a 'teat', which will reach well back into his mouth. As a result the tongue is unable to 'anchor' the 'teat', which then slips in and out of the baby's mouth as he sucks, exposing the nipple to friction, similar to a heel in an ill-fitting new shoe.

The best treatment for sore/cracked nipples lies ideally in prevention. This can be achieved by ensuring a successful beginning to breastfeeding, by slotting in a period of 'quality time' to teach and help the mother to achieve and recognize correct positioning. However, if the nipples have become sore, the immediate treatment must again be to check and correct positioning of the baby at the breast (see Chapter 9). A sore nipple can improve during a feed, when the baby has been enabled to latch on correctly (Fisher and Saunders, personal communication).

It has recently been suggested that if the soreness of the cracked nipple is due to a combination of dry skin and friction, some non-irritating ointment could be helpful (Sharp, 1992).

However the use of such an ointment must go hand in hand with attention to correct positioning. There is nothing that will accelerate the healing of a nipple that is continually being damaged.

If the pain during breastfeeding is severe and expert help is unavailable, a short period of resting the nipple may be indicated. During this time milk will have to be expressed, either by hand or by gentle mechanical expression. Sometimes expressing with a pump causes further pain/damage.

A survey of breastfeeding practices undertaken by the National Perinatal Epidemiology Unit in Oxford found that 32 different methods were being used to help heal nipple damage (Garforth and Garcia, 1989). This highlighted not only just how common nipple trauma is, but also the inconsistency of advice that mothers could receive if there was no clear understanding of the underlying cause which leads to this problem. In spite of the lack of research based evidence on which to base the practice, some women may want to use some other treatment, e.g. ointments or sprays, and their wishes should be respected. The midwife should ensure that the cause of the problem is also tackled and that the mother's self-selected treatment will do no damage, even though it may do no good.

Short frenulum (tongue-tie)

This can sometimes be the cause of sore nipples. In most cases the baby can feed without causing pain, but the mother may need help to get the attachment exactly right - a few millimetres may make a difference.

If the tongue is restrained to the point where the baby is unable to get his tongue far enough over his lower gum to reach the lactiferous sinuses, even with skilled help, the baby should be referred to a paediatric surgeon for assessment.

Thrush/Candidiasis/Monilia infection

Thrush, as a cause of sore nipples or acute breast pain during and following a feed, has occurred more frequently in the last few years (L'Strange, 1994; personal

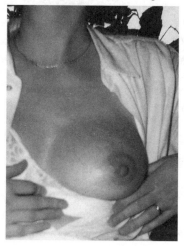

communication). A woman who has been treated with antibiotics is more vulnerable to this infection (Amir, 1991). The fungal organism, Candida Albicans, is more commonly known as the cause of monilial vulvovaginitis in women. In babies it may cause oral thrush, presenting as white buccal patches and white tongue, or persistent sore buttocks with or without a tongue lesion.

A mother with an inflamed area around the areola due to thrush

During a feed the thrush is likely to spread to the grooves on the surface of the nipple which are ideal places for the candida organisms, which thrive on milk, to grow and multiply (Lawrence, 1994). The infection may spread outwards from sore nipples on to the areola and sometimes beyond. The skin becomes slightly raised, itchy, shiny and red. Migration of the candida into the lactiferous ducts is signified by acute, deep pain in the breast during and particularly after the end of a feed, lasting several minutes.

Successful treatment for thrush has become more difficult as some candida organisms have changed and become resistant to some of the treatments mentioned below. The drugs prescribed are generally local anti-fungal preparations for mother and baby. Commonly, nystatin suspension or Micanozole for the baby's mouth and the mother's nipples/areola. (Clotrimazole should be avoided, as the ointment base may itself cause skin irritation on the nipple). For a vaginal infection antifungal pessaries would be indicated, when a partner may also have to be treated to prevent possible re-infection.

Systemic treatment may be prescribed if local treatment fails to clear the infection. Lawrence advises rigorous treatment to prevent a chronic condition from developing. Treatment may have to be prolonged for up to one month to ensure the infection has cleared completely (Saunders, 1994, personal communication).

As reinfection can occur very easily, the mother should be advised about attention to personal hygiene, including hand washing, the use of paper towels, changing disposable breast pads with each feed and the wearing of cotton panties and bras which can be washed at high temperature.

Engorgement of the breasts

Two to four days following the birth the breasts undergo two changes - the blood supply increases and the uninhibited prolactin stimulates the cells of Acini to produce milk, whether the baby is breastfed or not. This is accompanied by venous congestion and the breasts become full and feel heavy and warm. Frequently the mother's temperature rises slightly.

Ideally the mother should be forewarned and know what to expect when the milk comes in. In particular she should know that the fullness and heaviness of the breasts is normal, and that provided the baby feeds well and 'empties' the breasts of milk, the fullness will subside within 24 - 48 hours.

This normal physiological event can develop into an iatrogenic problem. *Engorgement of the breasts,* when they become tense, full, tender and hot. Engorgement affects the whole breast, and often both breasts unlike mastitis. White (1992) found engorgement to be the second most common reason for giving up breastfeeding in the first six days after the birth.

Engorgement is a common and largely preventable condition which may occur as a result of:

- a delay in starting to breastfeed (or express milk)
- poor positioning of the baby at the breast
- restriction of both the frequency and duration of feeding
- all of which result in inadequate 'emptying' of the breasts.

The mother should be aware that:

- Nature is generous and the supply of milk may temporarily exceed the baby's need

- the baby may thus be satisfied with one side at a time leaving the second side uncomfortable until the next feed

- the pressure inside the breasts may flatten the nipple making it more difficult for the baby to attach well

- red areas appearing on the breast are a warning sign of inflammation developing due to stasis.

Relieving the discomfort:

- a well supporting bra should be worn between feeds to elevate the heavy breasts

- cold packs applied to the breasts may help to reduce the oedema and swelling

- applying warmth can be soothing and helps the milk to flow. This is most easily achieved by either applying warm flannels with the breasts whilst leaning over a basin, or sitting in a bath. Alternatively the mother could spray the breasts with warm water in a shower

- the mother can be taught to express some milk manually between feeds to relieve discomfort and/or to soften the area behind the nipple, if it is difficult to latch the baby to the breast (see Chapter 9).

- the baby should be given unrestricted access to the breast

- attention should be paid to the attachment of the baby at each feed.

Severe engorgement can ensue if this situation is not resolved. The breasts become rock-hard and oedematous due to additional lymphatic congestion. This is very painful and the mother feels hot, shivery and quite ill (Minchin, 1985).

Apart from the acute discomfort, severe engorgement has two adverse effects on breastmilk production:

i)   the distended alveoli exert back pressure and flatten the milk producing cells with the consequent suppression of milk production (Dawson, 1935).

ii)   an autocrine inhibitory factor in breastmilk exerts a local inhibitory effect on further milk synthesis (Woolridge, 1993).

In addition to the above treatments, a mild analgesic may be necessary (Lawrence, 1989). Milk expression may be difficult. Help with positioning the baby and getting the baby to suckle is the surest way of resolving the condition.

Application of cabbage leaves to treat severe engorgement

In 1988, Rosier described a treatment for severely engorged breasts which consisted of the application of cold (refrigerated) cabbage leaves to the breasts. These were applied at two hourly intervals until the oedema was substantially reduced. The milk flow was reported to improve within hours and the milk supply adjusted satisfactorily. It was suggested the milk supply might be reduced if the treatment continued for too long, and that it was advisable to discontinue the treatment as soon as the oedema had subsided.

More recently, a randomized controlled study (Nicodem, 1993) examined the concept of preventing engorgement with the prophylactic application of cabbage leaves. The mothers applied cold cabbage leaves to the breasts (from approximately 72 hours after delivery) for the next four feeds, leaving them in place until they reached body temperature, about 20 minutes (A hole was cut in the leaves to allow the nipples to be kept dry).

The women in the experimental group reported less engorgement but this trend was not statistically significant.

However, a questionnaire completed by the mothers at six weeks postpartum found the mean duration of exclusive breastfeeding to be longer in the experimental group. It was not possible to determine whether this was due to the cabbage leaf application or was secondary to the reassurance and attention that these mothers had received, perhaps resulting in improved confidence and self esteem.

The application of cabbage leaves appears to do no harm but whether they are actually helpful remains to be established.

Blocked ducts

A blocked duct obstructs the flow of milk, which builds up behind the blockage and forms a hard lump. The lump is likely to be tender. If the blockage is unrelieved it may progress to mastitis (inflammation) as milk escapes into the surrounding tissue causing reddening of the overlying skin. Inflammatory products may get into the circulation and cause a flu-like reaction with an elevated temperature (Stanway, 1983).

The *causes* may be:

• the repeated inadequate emptying of a lobe, as a result of less than optimal positioning

• pressure of a badly fitting bra on a specific area, especially if worn at night

Prevention

Ensuring that the baby is correctly attached at the breast, so that all areas of the breast are equally and effectively drained.

When the baby has come off the breast spontaneously, the mother should palpate it, to ensure all areas are soft, before offering the second side to the baby. If not, the baby could continue feeding on the first side, if he is willing, with renewed attention to the positioning.

Treatment

The aim is to clear the lump as soon as it is detected to prevent this blockage from developing into mastitis by:

- improving the positioning of the baby at the breast.

- changing the feeding position of baby or mother (see Chapter 9 for different positions) so that the mother can position the baby more effectively.

- beginning the feed on the affected side, so that it is exposed to the vigour of the hungry baby's sucking. This procedure may have to be repeated at the next feed. Some milk may need to be expressed from the second breast if it feels uncomfortable i.e. if the baby is satisfied with one side only.

- gentle massage of the lump towards the nipple while the baby is feeding, followed by gentle pressure on the firm site with extended fingers as the baby suckles may help to withdraw the milk. The mother can usually feel the firm lobe becoming softer.

If the lump is not resolving the mother could try:

- applying warmth to the affected area to help the milk to flow and then gently massaging the lumpy area towards the nipple with the flat of the fingers, when the baby starts to feed.

- expressing her breasts after the feed.

White spot – Corpora amylacea

Some women report the presence of discrete lumps in their breastmilk, i.e. it appears particulate when expressed.

These white granules appear to be caused by the aggregation and fusion of casein micelles to which further materials become added. This may become hardened with the addition of hydroxyapatite, a mineral containing calcium phosphate and chloride (or fluoride) (Cowie, 1980; ALCA News, 1992).

This hardened lump may obstruct a milk duct as it slowly makes its way down to the nipple, where it may be removed by the baby during a feed (Hoyle, 1982) or expressed manually (ALCA News, 1992; Purves, 1982; Browne, 1982; Gottleib, 1982).

Some mothers describe strings or lengths of fatty looking material (Minchin, 1985). This may be similar to some of the material that could be expressed in Bertand's study (1991), and may be the origin of the idea that ducts could be blocked by thickened or inspissated milk.

Yet others report the end of the duct (at the nipple) being occluded by a 'blister', 'scab' or overgrowth of epithelium (Lodge, 1982; Taylor, 1982; Kennedy, 1982; Brown, 1982; Fisher, 1982), which can be removed with the fingernails, a rough flannel or with the aid of a blunt needle (Brown. 1982).

Unfortunately, blockages of this sort tend to recur but once the woman knows what they are and how to deal with them, mastitis can be avoided.

Mastitis

Signs and symptoms of mastitis rarely occur in the first week of lactation.

The signs and symptoms are:

- the mother feels ill with flu-like symptoms and a raised temperature (>38.4 degrees)

- the breast is painful and hot with an inflamed, localized wedge-shaped area over one lobe of the breast (Niebyl, 1978).

A distinction can be made between non-infective and infective mastitis, with a ratio of 50:50 between the two (RCM, 1991).

Non-infective mastitis

Causes are often the same as for a blocked duct, that is:

- the repeated inadequate emptying of a lobe, as a result of less than optimal positioning

- pressure of a badly fitting bra on a specific area, especially if worn at night

In addition:

- sudden trauma to the breast, such as the knee, elbow or foot of an older child

- an abrupt change in feeding pattern, such as the child suddenly sleeping through the night.

Prevention and management are the same as for a blocked duct (i.e. improved drainage of the breast). Antibiotics are not required.

However, the difference between this condition and infective mastitis is not always easy to distinguish clinically, culturing milk samples takes several days, and as a result antibiotics are frequently given for both conditions.

In 1984 Thomsen demonstrated that counting the bacteria and leucocytes in a sample of breastmilk would allow rapid differentiation and suggested the following criteria:

$<10^6$ leucocytes/ml $<10^3$ bacteria/ml	continue breastfeeding - no treatment necessary
$<10^6$ leucocytes/ml $>10^3$ bacteria/ml	continue breastfeeding - then express breastmilk after the feed
$<10^6$ leucocytes/ml $<10^3$ bacteria/ml	continue breastfeeding -express breastmilk as before - give antibiotics

Vets faced with mastitis use leucocyte counts to assist their differential diagnosis and treatment (Ballek, 1979) and there is no reason why this facility should not be available in hospital laboratories, but to date there seems to have been little demand.

Infective mastitis

When this condition occurs, it presents itself rapidly (Lawrence, 1989) *and needs speedy treatment* to prevent the formation of an abscess. The most common causative organism being the staphylococcus aureus.

Predisposing factors

- progression from a blocked duct or non-infective mastitis which has not responded to treatment (Lawrence, 1994)
- ascending staphylococcal aureus infection from a cracked nipple (Niebyl, 1978).
- poor hygiene, in particular the failure to wash hands before feeding.

Management of mastitis

Mastitis needs medical attention and the prescription of a suitable antibiotic that does not preclude breastfeeding.

- Bed rest may be desirable while flu-like symptoms persist

- Breastfeeding must continue and every effort should be made to ensure effective milk removal

- Some mothers find moist warm compresses soothing, others prefer a cold compress

- The mother should maintain an adequate fluid intake

- Analgesics may be required.

Breast abscess

Delayed treatment for mastitis may result in the formation of an abscess (the delay might amount to only a matter of hours).

Conventional treatment:

- a surgical incision and drainage of the accumulated pus
- the insertion of a drainage tube may be necessary for 48 hours
- antibiotics will be required
- The baby should continue with breastfeeding unless pus drains from the nipple.

In a new treatment described by Dixon in 1988 an abscess was successfully treated by aspiration with a needle and syringe.

White nipple (nipple blanching)

This painful condition sometimes occurs in women who suffer from Reynaud's syndrome or other circulatory problems. Positioning of the baby at the breast should be checked as it is often triggered by trauma to the nipple. Helpful reported remedies include feeding in a warmer room and drinking tea (which contains the vaso-dilator theophylline) before the feed (RCM, 1991).

CHAPTER FIFTEEN

Breastfeeding 'on Demand' and Hypoglycaemia

The definition of neonatal hypoglycaemia or low blood sugar is a controversial issue. In 1988 Koh reviewed 36 major paediatric text books and found the definition, in terms of glucose concentration, to range from <1mmol/l to <2.5mmol/l for normal healthy term babies (Modal value 1.7mmol/l) (Koh et al, 1988).

For the same review, 178 paediatricians were approached for their definition of neonatal hypoglycaemia and this demonstrated an even wider variation, with values of glucose concentrations between <1mmol/l to 4mmol/l (Modal value 2mmol/l).

Midwifery textbooks also vary in their definition. Myles' *Textbook for Midwives* (1985) quotes 1.6mmol/l and Mayes' *Midwifery*, 7mmol/l (Sweet, 1988).

The CIBA Foundation discussion meeting convened to address the current status of the definition of significant hypoglycaemia concluded 'The rational definition is clearly not a specific value but a continuum of falling glucose levels... which may vary from one cause of hypoglycaemia or clinical circumstance to another' (Cornblath, 1990).

The treatment for hypoglycaemia described in textbooks hardly mentions the normal neonate. It invariably relates to babies 'at risk' such as:

a)   babies of diabetic mothers because of the possible over-production of insulin in the first hours of extra-uterine life

b)   small for gestation infants who suffer from lack of glycogen reserves.

Babies whose blood sugar *must* be monitored include:

- Babies of proved hyperinsulinism
- Babies who are small for gestational age
- Premature babies
- Babies with systemic illness
- Babies who suffered birth asphyxia and hypothermia (Hawdon, 1993).

Blood sugar concentrations following birth

During intra-uterine life the fetal blood sugar is similar to that of the mother (Heck, 1987). The adaptation of the newborn to extra uterine life, with the sudden deprivation of all nourishment, is a veritable miracle.

The child deals with this sudden deprivation of the blood glucose as the cord is cut by:

* inhibiting insulin secretion
* the utilisation of hepatic glycogen (Sperling, 1982).

Blood glucose levels are at their lowest about an hour following birth and then begin to rise, even if enteral feeds are withheld (Srinivasan et al, 1986). The baby has the ability to generate ketone bodies from the fatty acids released from adipose tissue as the blood glucose concentration falls, which then serves as alternative fuel for the brain.

Hawdon, commenting in 1993, felt that this early self-limiting period of hypoglycaemia could not be considered pathological and that measuring the blood glucose concentration of asymptomatic babies within the first two hours was of little practical value. Having studied the metabolic adaptation of term infants in the first postnatal week, she concluded that blood glucose concentrations below <2.6mmol/l recurred in many healthy babies during the first three days of life, particularly if they were breast and demand fed with long intervals between feeds (Hawdon, 1992). To compensate for this, healthy, breastfed term babies of normal weight initiate a marked ketogenic response to low blood glucose concentrations. Evidence from animal studies suggest that this response is protective of neurological function (Hawdon, 1993).

This does not mean that a sleeping baby can be left and ignored until it wakes! Every newborn baby is an 'unknown quantity' and deserves observation to ensure his colour is good and that respirations and temperature are normal.

Assessment of blood sugar concentrations

The assessment of blood sugar concentrations in the neonate is a very common procedure.

The methods most commonly used, BMstix or Dextrostix reagent strips, have been criticized (Aynsley Green, 1991) as they were initially developed for the assessment of the blood sugar of diabetic patients who are more likely to need warning of hyperglycaemia. It has been shown that results differ by ± 0.5mmols/l when compared with laboratory measurements, when these strips are used to try and detect hypoglycaemia (Aynsley Green, 1991).

Williams (1992) warned that this inherent inaccuracy could be compounded as a result of collecting inadequate volumes of blood on the reagent strip and/or failing to allow alcohol to evaporate from the skin after cleansing.

(The most accurate measurements of neonatal blood sugar are obtained with a bench top glucose electrode (YSI 2300 Stat Plus, YSI Ltd (Hawdon et al, 1993).

Breastfeeding guidelines and 'demand feeding'

Since 1989, the Joint Breastfeeding Initiative has encouraged the production of breastfeeding guidelines for Maternity units. One recommendation which seems to have caused difficulties is the concept of 'demand feeding' i.e. no set rules for either the number or the frequency of feeds (RCM, 1991).

Doubt is often expressed about a normal, healthy baby's ability to regulate his intake of nutrients. In other words, can a baby be left to decide how frequently, and more particularly how infrequently, he wants to feed?

The fear of brain damage (which may result from hypoglycaemia) and the lack of an agreed definition of hypoglycaemia in the normal neonate has contributed to difficulties in developing breastfeeding guidelines/policies in relation to demand feeding. It is often expected that a newborn baby will feed frequently, despite normative data which suggests that newborn babies usually feed infrequently in the first 24-48 hours (Inch and Garforth, 1989). Many variations of the 'permitted' duration of the interval between feeds exist and are built into guidelines according to local decisions. Individual health professionals working in the same clinical area may nevertheless have their own idea of what time limit is acceptable. These may vary from 3 hours to 4, 5, 6, 8 or 12 hours or 'until the baby wakes'.

Such conflicting advice can have several implications:

- Mothers may become confused because of inconsistent advice
- Mothers' confidence in their ability to breastfeed is likely to be undermined
- Unnecessary blood glucose estimations might be taken
- Additional fluids may be given.

Rajan (1994) urges that 'extra efforts should be made to overcome women's difficulties in ways that are tailored to their individual needs with paramount importance given to the roles of information, support and consistent advice'.

Curiously, neonatal hypoglycaemia received very little attention in the days when breastfeeding was restricted on the first and second day to respectively three and five minutes each side per feed (with no concessions made for a slow let down reflex!) and frequently no night feeds.

The 'sedated' baby

It is questionable whether babies of mothers who have had pethidine in labour should be left until they wake spontaneously for a feed. In relation to demand feeding and hypoglycaemia, one has to ask whether they can be considered to be 'normal'.

When pethidine is given *late* in the first stage of labour the problem is compounded because both mother and baby will feel sleepy after the birth, the ideal time for the first feed (Rajan, 1994).

In 1966 Kron observed that even low doses of sedative and analgesic drugs given to the mother in labour could alter the baby's responsiveness and compromise the crucial role of the baby in the initiation of lactation. To make matters worse, the baby will receive an additional dose of pethidine via the mother's breastmilk, which may further depress the central nervous system (Freeborn, 1980).

As previously discussed, these observations have been confirmed more recently by Righard (1990), who when studying the effects of labour ward routines, found that 25 of the 40 babies whose mothers had been given pethidine during labour made no spontaneous efforts to suckle during the first two hours following birth.

Clearly these facts must be taken seriously and allowances made when developing breastfeeding guidelines. Mothers who wish to breastfeed must be made aware of the effect that pethidine may have, so that they have some understanding of their own responses and of the behaviour of the baby following birth.

Summary
The following Aide Memoire is adapted from 'Prevention and management of neonatal hypoglycaemia' (Hawdon, Ward Platt, Aynsley Green, 1994).

- Demand feeding can be recommended for a healthy term baby of appropriate birth weight for gestational age.

- Transient hypoglycaemia is a normal phenomenon in the first two postnatal hours.

- After this period, blood glucose concentrations below 2.6mmol/l may recur in healthy babies.

- Healthy babies react with a ketogenic response to a lowering of the blood glucose concentration.

- Clinical assessments of a baby who sleeps for a long period are essential to ensure the baby's temperature and respirations are normal, the colour is good and there are no clinical signs of dehydration or hypoglycaemia.

- Supplementary feeds of water, dextrose or formula milk are contra-indicated for normal healthy neonates.

- Monitoring blood glucose concentrations in healthy, appropriately grown neonates are unnecessary and potentially harmful to parental well-being and the establishment of successful breastfeeding.

- If an assessment of the blood sugar concentration is deemed advisable a proper laboratory tests should be undertaken.

CHAPTER SIXTEEN

Jaundice and Breastfeeding

Physiological jaundice

Jaundice, the visible sign of a raised serum bilirubin level, is so common in babies between the ages of two to five days of age that it is often referred to as 'physiological jaundice'. It develops in nearly 50 per cent of all healthy babies born at term.

Bilirubin is one of the break-down products of the haem factor of haemoglobin. As the level of bilirubin in the blood rises, first the sclera, and then the face become slightly yellow, followed by yellowing of the body. Jaundice is seldom seen over the lower leg and tibia until the serum bilirubin rises approaches 250umols/l (Hey, 1995). As (unconjugated, fat-soluble) bilirubin is released into the bloodstream from the spleen, it is bound to an albumen molecule and transported to the liver. Here it is processed and conjugated into a water-soluble, non-toxic substance and excreted via the bile duct into the gut. In its unconjugated (fat-soluble) form, bilirubin is toxic to all cells, particularly brain cells, which cannot re-generate if they are destroyed by bilirubin deposits (Hansen, 1986). The level at which unconjugated bilirubin may do harm depends on a number of factors, including maturity, birth weight and the presence or absence of acidosis, hypoxia, hypoglycaemia, hypothermia or sepsis (Lawrence, 1994).

If a baby is very immature, very small or suffers from any of these conditions the timing of the first feed is very likely to be delayed as well as the infant's readiness to suckle.

For reasons which are poorly understood, the maximum safe level is lower in pre-term than in term babies, and lower in babies with haemolytic jaundice than with 'physiological' jaundice (Hey, 1995).

In physiological jaundice the serum bilirubin rises from birth to the third - fourth day, reaching an average level of 100umol/l. It then declines to reach adult levels (<15umols/l) by about the tenth or eleventh day (Robertson, 1993).

Physiological jaundice is the most commonly treated medical condition in otherwise healthy newborns (Osborn, 1984). Phototherapy is the recommended treatment if the serum bilirubin rises to above 14 - 15 mg/dl (239 - 257umol/l) and exchange transfusion if the level reaches 20mg/dl (342umol/l) (Oski, 1988). Hey maintains that there is only very weak evidence to support this very precise recommendation (Hey, 1995).

Jaundice which develops *during the first day* invariably has a pathological cause.

Main factors responsible for raising bilirubin levels

a)   The inability of the liver to deal with the amount of bilirubin produced by the normal catabolism of fetal red blood cells. These have a lifespan shorter than that of adult red cells, 90 days rather than 120 days, and are thus broken down at a more rapid rate. If this is faster than the liver can 'process' the breakdown products, bilirubin levels rise. This may be a consequence of prematurity, glucose-6-phosphate-dehydrogenase (G6PD) deficiency, glucuronyl transferase or other enzyme deficiency or because the cells are breaking down at an accelerated rate (see 'e' below).

b)   Decreased albumin binding, which may occur if the infant is pre-term, or is given drugs (such as aspirin or sulphonamide) which release bilirubin from its binding protein.

c)   Increased re-absorption of bilirubin from the meconium in the gut. This may be the result of restricted feeding, pyloric stenosis or other forms of intestinal obstruction. Meconium contains an accumulated amount of bilirubin deposited in the gut during intra-uterine life. If its expulsion is slow, conjugated bilirubin is re-converted to unconjugated bilirubin which can cross the gut wall and re-enter the blood stream, raising the bilirubin level (Lawrence, 1994).

d)   Calorie deprivation - The association between starvation and hyper bilirubinaemia has been noted in both humans and animals but the exact mechanism is unclear (Gartner and Lee, 1980).

e)   An abnormally rapid rate of red cell breakdown, due to blood incompatibility, sepsis or (rarely) congenital sphcrocytosis.

Normal haematological values of the infant		
Total blood volume	78-100 mls/kg body weight	
Red blood cells	at birth:	5.8 million/ml
	at 14 days:	5.1 million/ml
	at 3 months:	3-4 million/ml
Haemoglobin	at birth:	18.4gm/100ml
	80 per cent is fetal haemoglobin	
	at 14 days:	16.8gm/100ml
	at 10 weeks	12.0gm/100
1gm haemoglobin produces 34 mg (598.5umol/l) bilirubin		

(Partly adapted from Klaus and Farnaroff. Care of the high-risk neonate, W.B. Saunders Co. Philadelphia, 1979)

Incidence of jaundice in breastfed babies

In a review of 12 studies Schneider (1986) found a considerably higher incidence of moderate jaundice (>204mmols/l) in breastfed infants compared to infants who were bottle fed.

	Number of jaundiced infants with >204umol/l bilirubin
Number of breastfed infants (3,997)	514
Number of bottle fed infants (4,255)	172

(Adapted from Schneider, A.P. (1986). 'Breastmilk jaundice in the newborn' *JAMA* , 255 (23): 3270-3274.)

The above study does not give details on the method of breastfeeding e.g. *when* breastfeeding was initiated or whether *demand feeding* was practised.

In the same year Maisels (1986) found that 12 per cent of breastfed babies and five per cent of bottle fed babies had a peak bilirubin in excess of 194umol/l, confirming an earlier, UK study (Wood, 1979). Maisels' study demonstrated that breastfed babies not only tended to have higher peak bilirubin values but also remained jaundiced for a longer time.

A recent study (Salariya, 1993) compared the level of jaundice in breastfed babies who were demand fed, with artificially fed babies and babies who started to breastfeed but changed to artificial feeding before five days of age or prior to the passage of the baby's first yellow stool. The results showed that although the breastfed babies had their first feed earlier than the artificially fed babies there was a significant increase in the proportion of breastfed babies who developed jaundice when compared with the babies who were artificially fed or those who changed from breast to artificial feeding. Breastfed babies also took significantly longer to pass the first yellow stool and lost more mean percentage weight when compared to the two other groups. The author recommends that midwives be alert to assist the breastfeeding woman who is experiencing difficulties in the first two postnatal days in order to try and reduce the proportion of babies who develop neonatal jaundice.

Feeding type	Breast % (No=63)	Artificial % (No=51)	Breast to artificial % (No=36) *
Level of jaundice			
None	58 (37)	82 (42)	64 (23)
Mild * *	24 (15)	16 (8)	28 (10)
Severe * * *	17 (11)	2 (1)	8 (3)

*   initially breastfed, but changed to artificial feeding before 5 days
* *   5 - 11.9mg% (85.5 - 203.5umol/l)
* * *   12 - 19.9mg% (205.2 - 340.3umol/l)

Incidence of jaundice
(Adapted from Salariya, E.M, Robertson, C.M., 1993)

Breastfeeding practices which influence the level of jaundice

Delayed first feed and infrequent feeding

A low intake of colostrum, due to rigid, infrequent early feeding policies has been implicated as a cause of jaundice in breastfed infants. Denying the infant colostrum delays the clearance of meconium (Gartner, 1980), which in turn may cause serum bilirubin levels to rise (De Carvalho, 1982).

This relationship between the delayed passage of meconium and jaundice was already observed by Condie in 1859, when he wrote: 'Generally speaking (Icterus neonatorum)...has appeared to be connected with the want of a free evacuation of the meconium'.

A distinction needs to be made between not restricting feed frequency and encouraging frequent feeds. Whilst restricting feeds may be deleterious to breastfeeding and SBR levels, (De Carvahlo, 1982, 1983), deliberately increasing the frequency of the feeds beyond the demands of the healthy infant, has been shown to be of no benefit, either in terms of SBR levels or weight gain (Maisels, 1994).

Type of feeding - breast versus formula

When comparing the amount of stool passed by breastfed and bottlefed babies, Salaryia (1993) found that the latter excreted 82g in three days, which was 24g more than that passed by breastfed babies.

The colour of the breastfed baby's stool takes longer to change from black to yellow than does the stool of an artificially fed baby. Salaryia also found that breastfed babies lost more mean percentage weight when compared with both the artificially fed babies and the breastfed group who changed to artificial feeding.

Feeding type	Breast % (No=63)	Artificial % (No=51)	Breast to artificial % (No=36)
Time to pass first stool			
<2 days	5 (3)	16 (8)	11 (4)
3 days	27 (17)	49 (25)	14 (5)
4 days	38 (24)	10 (5)	28 (10)
5 days	13 (8)	18 (9)	8 (3)
>5 days	17 (11)	8 (4)	39 (14)

(From Salariya and Robertson, 1993)

Salariya (1993b) developed a stool colour comparator to demonstrate the transition process of stool colour from meconium to yellow. Midwives at the study hospital used the comparator in the postnatal ward. It was introduced to correlate stool colour-change timing, along with other criteria, to determine the quality of early baby feeding, especially breastfeeding in the first five days.

It is clearly important for midwives to be ready and able to assist the breastfeeding woman who is experiencing difficulties in the first two postnatal days so that the normal physiological processes of both mother and baby are not disturbed. At the same time, it is, in Hey's view:

> 'a sad indictment of the medical approach to normality that we now define "normality" by the performance of the average bottle fed baby. As a result we tend to look upon the low enterohepatic recirculation of bilirubin that accompanies the frequent, incompletely digested stool of the bottlefed baby as being more normal than the continuing milk jaundice caused by the efficient gastrointestinal performance of the breastfed baby.' (Hey, 1995).

Jaundice, breastfeeding and supplementary fluids

The giving of water (or dextrose) to babies with jaundice does nothing to lower peak bilirubin levels (Nicoll, 1982; De Carvalho, 1982; Dahms, 1973). This should come as no surprise, as unconjugated serum bilirubin is fat soluble, not water-soluble.

Indeed this practice may even cause serum bilirubin levels to rise, by reducing the intake of milk and thus the rate at which meconium is evacuated (Nicoll, 1982; De Carvalho, 1982; Jesuru, 1979; Kuhr and Paneth, 1982).

If the baby is breastfed, filling his stomach with water is likely to reduce the number of feeds he takes and thus interrupt the establishment of lactation. Women whose babies are given additional fluids are much more likely to stop breastfeeding in the first six weeks than those whose babies receive nothing but breastmilk (White, 1992).

Most local breast-feeding guidelines recommend that 'breastfed babies should not normally be offered complementary feeds or water'. In one area, where this guideline was in place, it was found that 42 per cent of health professionals were still giving water and 8 per cent still giving dextrose either frequently or very frequently - in total disregard for the recommendation made in the guidelines (Beeken, 1992).

From the response to questions posed at breastfeeding study days I have attended during the last five years, regarding the giving of water, it is clear that this practice is commonplace. Nationally 45 per cent of breastfed babies are still receiving fluids other than breastmilk whilst in hospital, often in defiance of local guidelines.

Prevention (and treatment) of 'physiological' jaundice

- Putting the baby to the breast in the labour ward to encourage early passage of meconium.

- Ensuring that the baby is well positioned at the breast, to make the colostrum available.

- Offering the breast frequently, particularly if the baby has become jaundiced i.e. rousing the baby when he is just stirring, rather than hoping that he will sleep a little longer.

- Assisting the mother with breastfeeding, particularly if the baby is sleepy (This should be anticipated, if the mother has had pethidine in labour).

- Observing stools for changing colour from meconium to a changing then yellow stool. If there is any delay in the change of colour, this should prompt a re-assessment of the mother's feeding technique.

- *Avoid giving water or dextrose fluids*

Does jaundice need treating?

Both the age of the baby and the total serum bilirubin level need to be taken into consideration when deciding whether to treat jaundice in a term baby.

Newman (1992) considered the risk associated with high bilirubin levels in otherwise well, term infants to be small and the benefits of treatment, if any, likely to be small as well and possibly increasing the risk.

He also deplored the temporary interruption of breastfeeding that often accompanied such treatment, as it so often led to the abandonment of breastfeeding.
Kemper (1989) found that mothers consider jaundice a serious illness and that this concern tended to persist for at least a month, during which time the risk of terminating breastfeeding was substantially increased.

Hey (1995) is of the opinion that 'Jaundice probably only calls for medical intervention, in the absence of haemolytic disease, in the one term baby in a thousand...in whom the levels reach 430umol/l'.

The breastfed baby who undergoes phototherapy treatment

Should phototherapy be considered necessary, it should not interfere with breastfeeding. Robertson (1993) emphasises that babies should be allowed out from phototherapy to breastfeed, unless the serum bilirubin is approaching exchange level.

Babies receiving phototherapy tend to lose more fluid than they would otherwise. They may be drowsy as a consequence of their raised bilirubin. Extra attention should thus be paid to the quality of the feeds. The baby should be offered the breast at least every four hours. If he feeds well, nothing further need be done. If he is too sleepy to feed, the mother should be shown how to express her milk by hand or by pump, and this should be offered to the baby.

Separating mother and baby for phototherapy alone serves no useful purpose, it merely increases the stress levels in the mother (as measured by urine cortisol levels) and increases the likelihood that she will stop breastfeeding (Elander, 1986).

Breastmilk or late-onset jaundice

In approximately two to four per cent of breastfed babies, jaundice does not resolve towards the end of the first week but increases into the second and third week with a serum bilirubin, which if unchecked, can rise to above 342umol/l (Lawrence, 1994). The jaundice may even continue into the second and third month (Auerbach, 1987). On examination the baby is well and there is no correlation with weight loss or gain and stools are normal. Breastmilk jaundice is associated with the milk of a particular mother and will occur with each of her pregnancies in varying degrees, depending on each infants ability to conjugate bilirubin (Lawrence, 1994). The cause is a yet unknown factor present in breastmilk. Robertson (1993) writes that '...there are many theories but there is still no consensus.' Providing the baby is well and the serum bilirubin level remains within acceptable limits no action needs to be taken.

However if the jaundice persists for more than three weeks' particularly if the stools are persistently pale and putty coloured rather than yellow or green, biliary atresia should be excluded (Hey, 1995).

Diagnosis and treatment

Provided that this one condition is not overlooked, Hey maintains that 'no important treatable condition will be missed by dispensing with further investigations when prolonged jaundice is encountered in an otherwise vigorous and thriving breastfed term baby'.

The diagnosis of breastmilk jaundice could be confirmed by suspending breastfeeding for 24 -48 hours or alternating breast with formula feeding and monitoring the serum bilirubin levels (Newman, 1992). During this interruption of breastfeeding the baby would need to be fed with either banked breastmilk or formula milk, while the mother would need to express her milk to keep up the supply. Breastfeeding could then resume after the diagnostic fall in serum bilirubin level had taken place. It generally rises again once breastfeeding is recommenced, but not to the previous level (Auerbach, 1987).

Hey considers this diagnostic suspension of breastfeeding to be quite unnecessary and argues that taking the baby off the breast merely leads the mother to feel that she is harming her baby in some way. If serum bilirubin levels are causing concern, a short course of low dose phototherapy is more effective than two days of formula feeds (Hey, 1995).

CHAPTER SEVENTEEN

Breastfeeding Initiatives in the United Kingdom

The Joint Breastfeeding Initiative

In 1980 and 1985, the Office of Population Censuses and Surveys (OPCS) carried out their second and third investigation into 'Infant Feeding' in the United Kingdom (Martin, 1982, 1988).

Postal questionnaires were sent to 6,498 women in 1980 and 8154 women in 1985 six weeks after they gave birth. The women were sent a second questionnaire four months after the birth and a final one at nine months.

These surveys established that in England and Wales:

- in 1980 the breastfeeding rate at birth was 67 per cent
- in 1980 the breastfeeding rate at six weeks was 42 per cent
- in 1985 the breastfeeding rate at birth was 65 per cent
- in 1985 the breastfeeding rate at six weeks was 40 per cent

By 1990, both rates had fallen by a further one per cent.

The decline over the six week period (which was the same in all three surveys), became known as 'The lost 25 per cent'.

Of the many findings in the 1985 survey, three were of particular concern to both health professionals and the lay breastfeeding organizations:

i)   There had been no improvement in the number of mothers who had stopped breastfeeding by six weeks, by comparison with the 1980 survey

ii)   Many women were stopping earlier than they would have liked because of problems, most of which appeared to have been either preventable or easily solved with good support

iii) Even though most women had sought help from a health professional when they had difficulties, their difficulties had not been resolved.

These findings became the catalyst which generated Government support for a four year project *The Joint Breastfeeding Initiative.*

The Government's involvement in supporting breastfeeding had hitherto been limited to:

a)   publishing expert reports concerning infant feeding, which were then adopted as Government policy (see chapter 3). (These reports invariably stressed the benefits and superiority of breastfeeding.)

b)   financial support which had been given to voluntary breastfeeding organizations on an annual basis.

In 1988, Mrs. Edwina Currie, the then Minister of Health, agreed that in spite of the long-standing record of the Government of promoting good infant feeding practices, more needed to be done. She turned to the voluntary breastfeeding groups to support an initiative in conjunction with all health professional organizations.

On 18th October 1988, The Joint Breastfeeding Initiative (JBI) was launched at a symposium at the King's Fund Centre in London, with representatives of these organizations from all over country.

A multi-disciplinary National Steering Group was set up, chaired by a breastfeeding counsellor from the National Childbirth Trust, Mrs. Barbara Henry. Dora Henschel, a senior health professional, was appointed by the minister as National Co-ordinator. The Steering group was made up of representatives from all the health professional organizations whose members were involved in some way with breastfeeding mothers, as well as representatives of the three voluntary breastfeeding support groups (The representatives were chosen by their own organization).

The JBI was a new venture with more direct input by the Department of Health, who also sent observers to attend the meetings of the National JBI Steering Group.

One of the main objectives of the JBI was to encourage District Health Authorities (DHAs) to set up local breastfeeding working groups. Like the National Group, the local JBI groups were to be composed of health professionals, mainly midwives and health visitors and local breastfeeding counsellors from the National Childbirth Trust, La Leche League and the Association of Breastfeeding Mothers. Participation from other health professions such as general practitioners, paediatricians, dieticians, school nurses and community medical and health education officers ultimately varied from group to group.

Four years after the launch of the JBI, 141 groups had been set up, while some DHAs/ NHS Trusts were still working towards starting a group. The enthusiasm of the groups, and their commitment to improving the breastfeeding situation, was heartening.

A booklet published by the Department of Health 'The National Breastfeeding Initiative. Supporting and Promoting Breastfeeding: A National Initiative' suggested that the groups might:

a)   review the local breastfeeding guidelines and revise them as needed.

b)   ensure that local policies are known to all concerned with the breastfeeding mother and those who give her support.

c)   enable these policies to be put into action.

d)   provide a means of monitoring these policies.

e)   review the need for education of health care staff, other professionals, especially teachers and the public at large.

f)   collaborate with other bodies to meet local educational needs.

g)   raise public awareness of breastfeeding as the best way of feeding babies.

At the end of the four year period of the JBI, a questionnaire was sent to the Chair of each local breastfeeding working group to find out how many of these suggestions they had taken up.

It was found, in order of prevalence, that:

*   the last suggestion, *raising public awareness,* had received most support. This was possibly because of the introduction of the national '*Breastfeeding Awareness Week*', which has remained annual event since 1990.

*   the first suggestion, *development or up-dating of local breastfeeding guidelines,* was second, with 4/5th of DHAs having up-dated their guidelines on research-based information (RCM, 1991).

*   suggestion 'e', *reviewing the need for breastfeeding education,* had been implemented in a 'patchy' way. In most DHAs some in-service training had been given but only ten District Health Authorities had actually introduced training for all midwifery staff, following the introduction of new guidelines. The length of the training varied from 2 - 28 hours.

The importance of in-service training for staff when new guidelines are being implemented cannot be stressed enough. If trained staff do not understand the basis of the guidelines they will probably ignore them and old-fashioned routines and conflicting advice are likely to continue. It is still the case, sadly, that 'despite sound, research-based guidelines (RCM, 1991) on which midwives can base their practice, there remains a theory-practice gap' (Parker, 1994).

Other activities instigated by local Breastfeeding Working Groups were collection of local breastfeeding statistics e.g. rates of breastfeeding at:

*   birth
*   on discharge from hospital
*   and/or from midwifery care
*   at 4/6/8 weeks and/or 4 months

- organization of breastfeeding study days/workshops
- designing breastfeeding posters/leaflets
- introducing a telephone breastfeeding help line

A JBI newsletter was published quarterly and several copies of each issue were sent to the Chair of all the local working groups as well as the Chair of all the Maternity Services Liaison Committees.

Overall, perhaps the main achievement of the JBI, in the four years of its existence, was that it raised the profile of breastfeeding.

Its importance was acknowledged in the Government publication 'The Health of the Nation' (The Secretary of State for Health, 1992) in which it was proposed that 'the Government set up a National working group to help identify and take forward action to increase the proportion of infants breastfed, both at birth and at six weeks'.

National Breastfeeding Working Group

In March 1993, the *National Breastfeeding Working Group* had its first meeting. Its members, which this time included officers from the Department of Health with a senior officer as chairman, were all appointed by the Department of Health.

The Group's terms of reference were:

> 'To co-ordinate the next stages in a programme of action to facilitate breastfeeding, building on the achievements of the Joint Breastfeeding Initiative'.

With financial support from the Department of Health, the Group maintained the Breastfeeding Awareness Week and supported the existing (JBI) Breastfeeding Groups with their local efforts in that week. It also relaunched the newsletter in an attempt to keep the local groups in touch. In June 1995 the working group was wound up.

In May 1994, the Department of Health funded two fact-finding days as part of an Initiative to improve the training of health professionals. The purpose of this was to provide a basis for the production of a new training package 'Invest in Breast Together', (Kendall, 1995) a joint venture between the Royal College of Midwives and the Health Visitors Association. This learning pack has been developed to train effective breastfeeding trainers.

In May 1995 the National Breastfeeding Working Group completed and the Department of Health published:

1.   *Breastfeeding: A Summary of Educational Resources*

2.   *Breastfeeding: Good Practice, Guidance to the NHS*

During the two years and three months that the NBWG was in existence, the Department continued to support the annual National Breastfeeding Awareness Week, held during the months of May.

On May 26, 1995, Baroness Cumberledge announced the establishment of a National network of eight Regional Breastfeeding Co-ordinators, who will meet twice a year under the chairmanship of Mrs Cynthia Rickitt (formerly Head of Midwifery Services, Sunderland). The voluntary organizations will also be invited to send a representative. No further information is available at present (July, 1995).

At its first meeting, the group had agreed to work in partnership with the *UNICEF/ WHO 'Baby Friendly Initiative'*.

The initiative was developed following a Joint Statement of WHO and UNICEF (1989) entitled: 'Protecting, promoting and supporting breastfeeding: the special role of maternity services'.

It suggests the actions that can be taken by a hospital to achieve ten steps that lead to successful breastfeeding with regard to:

- policy and staff training
- structure and functioning of services
- health education
- aspects to be considered on discharge from hospital.

(WHO, 1989)

The 'Ten Steps to Successful Breastfeeding' were jointly formulated in 1989 by WHO/ UNICEF and form the basis of the Baby friendly Initiative (see Appendix II).

In August 1990 the WHO/UNICEF policy makers met in Florence to consider 'Breastfeeding in the 1990s: A Global Initiative'. As a result of this meeting the 'Innocenti Declaration' was formulated and adopted by participants of the meeting (UNICEF, 1990) (see Appendix III).

This Declaration calls for a permanent place for breastfeeding on every national agenda through the appointment of a multi-sectoral national breastfeeding committee and a national co-ordinator.

In June 1991, the 'Baby Friendly Hospital Initiative' (BFHI) was launched at the International Pediatric Association Conference in Ankara to take these statements and declarations forward.

The Baby Friendly Hospital Initiative aims to:

- recognize achievements of hospital facilities whose programmes encourage breastfeeding

- stimulate similar programmes in hospitals which have less than optimal support to breastfeeding (WHO/UNICEF, 1992a-c).

Some of its objectives are to:

*   enable mothers to make an informed choice on how to feed their newborns
*   support the initiation of breastfeeding
*   promote exclusive breastfeeding up to four - six months

The UNICEF/WHO Baby Friendly Initiative UK

In September 1991 the declaration was adopted by the World Summit for Children held in New York, in which the United Kingdom participated.

In March 1992, Mr Robert Smith, Director of UNICEF UK, invited representatives from organizations interested in breastfeeding to a round table discussion 'with a view to launching the Initiative in the UK in the most effective way'. A total of 14 health professional and 14 non-professional organizations responded and met to discuss the way forward in the UK. Multi-disciplinary working groups were set up with the ultimate aim to prepare an action plan for 'BFHI UK'.

A Director, Dr Michael W. Woolridge, was appointed to co-ordinate a strategy, which included the preparation and the publication of a 'Mother's Charter Protecting Breastfeeding Rights'. The BFHI UK was officially launched in November 1994.

One of the important actions of the BFHI is to encourage and assess hospitals interested in becoming designated as a 'Baby Friendly Hospital' by implementing the 'Ten Steps of Successful Breastfeeding' as follows.

Every Facility providing maternity services and care for newborn infants should:

1. Have a written breastfeeding policy that is routinely communicated to all health care staff.

2. Train all health care staff in skills necessary to implement this policy.

3. Inform all pregnant women about the benefits and management of breastfeeding.

4. Help mothers initiate breastfeeding within a half hour of birth.

5. Show mothers how to breastfeed and how to maintain lactation even if they should be separated from their infants.

6. Give newborn infants no food or drink other than breastmilk, unless *medically* indicated.

7. Practice rooming-in - allow mothers and infant to remain together 24 hours a day.

8. Encourage breastfeeding on demand.

9.   Give no artificial teats or pacifiers (also called dummies or soothers) to breastfeeding infants.

10.   Foster the establishment of breastfeeding support groups and refer mothers to them on discharge from the hospital or clinic.

Globally, nearly 1,000 hospitals have achieved this status. Most of these are in developing countries, the Philippines in particular.

In the industrialized world Sweden leads, with 20 of its 66 maternity facilities now designated as 'baby friendly' and with good support from its Government.

A package produced by the UK committee is now available and includes a Hospital Self-Appraisal Tool with which a hospital can begin the assessment process (WHO 1992a). If the hospital appears to measure up to the Global Criteria, it is formally assessed by a team from BFI UK, using the criteria set out in the Global Hospital Assessment Questionnaire and the Guide to Scoring the Hospital Assessment (WHO). This ensures that the assessment is the same in any setting, regardless of differences in culture and economy. To date (1995) four hospitals have been assessed.

Three of them have not yet achieved the rigorous criteria laid down and are working with the recommendations made for a repeat assessment.

Other areas with which the Initiative is concerned are:
•   Extending the Baby Friendly Initiative into the community
•   Training of health professionals
•   Informing, educating and empowering parents
•   Targeting policy makers
(Leaflet, UNICEF UK, 1994)

References

ACLA (1992). 'White spots (Corpora amylacea)'. *ALCA News*. December. Vol 3, No.3, pp.8-9.

Ajusi, J.D., Onyango, F.E., Mutanda, L.N. et. al. (1989). 'Bacteriology of unheated expressed milk stored at room temperature'. *East African Medical Journal*, 66: pp.381-87.

Akre, J. (1989). 'Infant feeding - the physiological basis'. Suppl., Vol. 67, *Bulletin of WHO*.

Alberti, K.G.M.M. (1993). 'Preventing insulin dependent diabetes mellitus'. *BMJ* 307: pp.435-36.

Alexander, J. (1990). 'Antenatal preparation of the breasts for breastfeeding', In: Alexander, J., Levy, V., Roch, S. (Eds). *Antenatal Care, A Research-Based Approach*. London: Macmillan.

Alexander, J., Grant, A.. Campbell, M. (1992). 'Randomized controlled trial of breast shells and Hoffman's exercises for inverted and non protractile nipples'. *BMJ*, 304: pp.1030-32.

American Academy of Pediatrics., Vitamin K Ad Hoc Task Force (1993). *Controversies Concerning Vitamin K and the Newborn*: 5, pp.1001-03.

Amir, L.H. (1991). 'Candida and the lactating breast: predisposing factors', *Journal Hum. Lact.*, 7: pp,177-81.

Aniansson, G. et. al. (1994). 'A prospective cohort study on breastfeeding and otitis media in Swedish infants'. *The Pediatric Infectious Disease Journal*, 13: pp.183-88.

Apple, R.D. (1987). *Mothers and Medicine: A Social History of Infant Feeding 1890 - 1950*. Madison: University of Wisconsin Press.

Applebaum, R. M. (1970). 'The modern management of successful breast-feeding'. *Pediatric Clinics of North America* 17; pp.203-25.

Arthur, P.G., Jones, T.J., Spruce, J., Hartmann, P.E. (1989). 'Measuring short-term rates of synthesis in breastfeeding mothers.' *Quarterly Journal of Experimental Physiology*, 74; pp.419-28.

Atherton, D.J., Sewell, M., Soothill, J.F., Wells, R.S., Chilvers, C.E.D. (1978). 'A double-blind controlled cross-over trial of an antigen-avoidance diet in atopic eczema', *Lancet*, i: pp.401-03.

Auerbach, K.G., Gartner, L.M. (1987). 'Breastfeeding and human milk: their association with jaundice in the neonate'. *Clin perinatol*; 14: pp.89-107.

Auerbach, K.G., Renfrew, M.J., Minchin, M. (1991). 'Infant feeding comparisons: A hazard to infant health?' *Journal of Human Lactation*; 7: pp.63-71.

Avoa, A. (1990). 'The influence of perinatal instruction about breastfeeding on neonatal weight'. *Pediatrics*; 86: pp.313-15.

Aynsley-Green, A. (1991). 'Glucose: a fuel for thought.' *Journal of Pediatr Child Health*; 27; pp.21-30.

Ball, J.A. (1987). *Reactions to Motherhood. The Role of Post-natal Care.* Cambridge: Cambridge University Press: pp.2, 95-104.

Ballek, J. (1979). 'Mastitis and milk cell counting' Department of Agriculture, Government of Victoria; Jan, Quoted in Minchin (1985).

Balmer, S.E., Hanvey, L.S., Wharton, B.A. (1994). 'Diet and faecal flora in the newborn: nucleotides' *Arch Dis Child*; 70: F137-F140.

Barger, J., Bull, P. (1987). 'A comparison of the bacterial composition of breastmilk stored at room temperature and stored in the refrigerator'. *Internat. J. Childbirth Ed.* pp.29-30.

Bates, C.J. (1985). 'Normal vitamin requirements in neonates and young children'. *Journal of Inherited Metabolic Diseases.* suppl 1, pp.8-12.

Bauchner, H., Leventhal, J.M., Shapiro, E.D. (1986). 'Studies of breastfeeding and infections. How good is the evidence'. *JAMA*; 256: pp.887-92.

Beeken, S., Waterston, T. (1992). 'Health service support of breastfeeding - are we practising what we preach?' *BMJ*; 305: pp.285-87.

Begley, C.M. (1993). *The Factors Affecting Duration of Breast-Feeding.* International Confederation of Midwives, 23rd international Congress, Vancouver.

Berkow, S., Freed, L., Hamosh, M. et. al. (1984). 'Lipases and lipids in human milk: effect of freeze-thawing and storage'. *Pediatr. Res.* 18: pp.1257-62.

Birch, E. et. al. (1993). 'Breastfeeding and optimal visual development'. *J. Ped. Opthalmol. Strab.* 30: pp.33-38.

Blanc, B. (1981). 'Biochemical aspects of human milk - comparison with bovine milk'. *World Rev. Nutr. Diet.* 36: pp.1-89.

Blomquist, H.K. et al. (1994). 'Supplementary feeding in the maternity ward shortens the duration of breastfeeding'. *Acta Paediatr.* 83: pp.1122-26.

Bourne, M.A. (1982). 'Sleep in the puerperium'. *Midwives Chronicle and Nursing Notes*: March: p.91.

Boyd, C., Sellers, L. (1982) *The British Way of Birth.* London: Pan Books.

Brackbill, Y. et al. (1974). 'Obstetric meperidine usage and assessment of neonatal status'. *Anaesthesiology*; 40: pp.116-20.

Brazelton, T. B. (1976). In: Marshall, H., Klaus, Kennell, J.H. (Eds). *Parent-Infant Bonding.* 2nd edition. St Louis: The C.V.Mosby Company. p.34.

Brown, L. (1982). 'Blocked ducts – revisited'. *New Generation.* 1 (4) pp.16-19.

Brown, L. (1992). 'Blocked ducts'. *New Generation.* 1 (1) pp.16-17.

Bruce, N.G., Khan, Z., Olsen, N.D.L. (1991). 'Hospital and other influences on the uptake and maintenance of breastfeeding: the development of infant feeding policy in a district. public health'. 105: pp.357-68.

Buescher, E.S., Pickering, L.K. (1986). 'Polymorphonuclear leucocytes in human colostrum and milk.' In: Howell, R.R., Morriss, R.H., Pickering, L.K. (Eds). *Human Milk in Infant Nutrition and Health.* Springfield II, Charles C Thomas.

Burr, M.L., Limb, S.E., Maguire, M.J., Amarah, L., Reldridge, B.A., Layzell, J.C.M., Merrett, T,G. (1993). 'Infant Feeding, wheezing, and allergy: a prospective study'. *Arch Dis Child*; 68: pp.724-28.

Butte et al. (1984). 'Feeding patterns of exclusively breast-fed infants during the first four months of life'. *Early Hum Dev*; 12: p.291.

Butte, N.E., Goldblum, R.M., Fehl, N.M., Loftin, K., Smith, E.O., Goldman, E.S. (1984). 'Daily ingestion of immunologic components in human milk during the first four months of life'. *Acta Paediatr. Scand.* 73, pp.296-301.

Campbell, H., Jones, I,G. (1993). *Scottish Needs Assessment Programme. Health Promotion Review. Breastfeeding in Scotland. Department of Public Health,* Fife Heath Board, Springfield House, Cupar KY15 5UP.

Carrington, R. (1965). 'The mammals, Netherlands', *Time-Life International:* p.37.

Carvalho, M., Robertson, S., Friedman, A., Klaus, M. (1983). 'Effect of frequent breastfeeding on early milk production and infant weight gain'. *Pediatrics,* 72 (3); pp.307-11.

Chandra, R.K. (1979). 'Prospective studies of the effect of breastfeeding in the incidence of infection and allergy', *Acta Paediatr Scand,* 68: pp.691-94.

Chappell, J.E., Clandinin, M.T., Kearney-Volpe, C. (1985). 'Trans fatty acids in human milk lipids: influence of maternal diet and weight loss'. *AM.J. Clin. Nutr.* 42: pp.49-56.

Cockburn, F. (1994). 'Neonatal brain and dietary lipids'. *Arch Dis Child.* 70: F1-F2.

Commission of the European Communities (1991). 'Commission directive on infant formulae and follow-on formulae'. *Official Journal of the European Communities.* No L 175/38.

Condie, D.F. (1859). *A Practical Treatise on the Diseases of Children,* 4th Edition, Philadelphia, Pensylvania: Blanchard and Lea.

Cornblath, M.D., Schwartz, R., Aynsley-Green, A., Lloyd, J.K. (1991). 'Hypo-glycaemia in infancy: The need for a rational definition. A CIBA foundation discussion meeting'. *Pediatrics;* 85: pp.834-37.

Corsini, G.U. (1971). 'Evidence for dopamine receptors in the human brain mediating sedation and sleep'. *Life Sciences* 20 (a): pp.1613-18.

Cowie, A.T., Forsyth, I.A., Hart, I.C (1980). 'Hormonal control of lactation'. *ALCA News,* 1992. Springer Verlag, Berlin.

Croucher, C., Azzopardi, ?. (1994). 'Compliance with recommendations for giving Vitamin K to newborn infants'. *British Medical Journal,* 308, pp.894-95.

Cumming, R.G., Klineberg, R.J. (1993). 'Breastfeeding and other reproductive factors and the risk of hip fractures in elderly women'; *Int J Epidemiol,* 22: pp. 684-91.

Cunningham, A.S. (1988). 'Studies of breastfeeding and infections. How good is the evidence? A critique of the answer from Yale.' *Journal of Human Lactation;* 4: pp.54-56.

Dahms, B.B., Klaus, A.N., Gartner, A.M., Klain, D.B., Soodalter, J. (1973). 'Breastfeeding and serum bilirubin values during the first four days of life'. *Journal Pediatr,* 83(6): pp.1049-54.

Daly, S. (1993). 'The short term synthesis and infant regulated removal of milk in lactating women'. *Experimental Physiology,* 78; pp.209-20.

Dawson, E.K. (1935). *Edinburgh Medical Journal;* 42: p.569.

De Carvalho, M., Hall, M., Harvey, D. (1981). 'Effects of water supple mentation on physiological jaundice in breastfed babies'. *Am J Dis Child* 56: pp.568-69.

De Carvalho, M., Klaus, M.H., Merkatz, R.B. (1982). 'Frequency of breastfeeding and serum bilirubin concentration'. *Am J Dis Child* 136: pp.737-38.

De Cavalho, M., Robertson, S., Friedman, A., Klaus, M. (1983). 'Effect of frequent breastfeeding on early milk production and infant weight gain'. *Pediatrics;* 72(3): pp.307-11.

De Chateau, P. et al. (1977). 'A Study of Factors Promoting and Inhibiting Lactation', *Develop Med Child Neurol;* 19: pp.575-84.

De Chateau, P., Wiberg, B. (1977). 'Long term effect on mother-infant behaviour of extra contact during the first hour post-partum'. *Acta Paediatrica Scandinavica* 66: pp.137-51.

Department of Health (1994). *Weaning and the Weaning diet. Report of the working group on the weaning diet of the committee on Medical aspects of food policy (COMA).* London: HMSO.

Department of Health and Social Security (1974) *Present Day Practice in Infant Feeding.* London: HMSO. (Reports on health and social subjects; No 9).

Department of Health and Social Security (1977). *The Composition of Mature Human Milk. DHSS Report on Health and Social subjects 12.* London: HMSO.

Department of Health and Social Security (1980). *Artificial Feeds for the young infant. DHSS Report on Health and Social Subjects 18.* London: HMSO.

Dewey, K.G., Heinig, M.J., Nommsen, L.A., Peerson, J.M., Lonnerdal, B. (1992). 'Growth of breast-fed and formula-fed Infants from 0 to 18 months: the DARLING study'. *Pediatrics,* 89(6); pp.1035-41.

Dick, G. (1976). 'The etiology of multiple sclerosis', *Proc R Soc Med,* 69: p.611.

Dixon, J.M. (1988). 'Repeated aspiration of breast abscess in lactating women'. *British Medical Journal.* 297: pp.1517-18.

Draper, G., McNinch, A. (1994). 'Vitamin K for neonates: the controversy'. *B.M.J.* 308, pp.867-68.

Drewett, R.F. et al. (1988). 'Pain during breastfeeding: The first three months postpartum'. *Journal of Reproductive and Infant Psychology,* 5: pp.183-86.

Drewett, R.F., Woolridge, M. (1981). 'Milk taken by human babies from the first and second breast'. *Physiology and Behaviour,* 26; pp.327-29.

Duncan ,B. et. al. (1993). 'Exclusive breastfeeding for at least four months protects against otitis media'. *Pediatrics,* 91 (5): pp.867-72.

Ebrahim, G.J. (1991). *Breastfeeding. The Biological Option.* 2nd Edn. ELBS with MacMillan.

Ebrahim, Z. (1995). 'Breastmilk immunology', *Journal Tropical Disease.* 41: pp.2-3.

Ekelund, H., Finnstrom, O., Gunnarskog, J., Kallen, B., Larson, Y. (1993). 'Administration of Vitamin K to newborn infants and childhood cancer'. *BMJ* 307: pp.89-91

Elander, G., Lindbeg, T. (1984). 'Short mother-infant separation during first week of life influences the duration of breastfeeding'. *Acta Paediatr Scan.* 73: pp.140-44.

Elander, G., Lindburg, T. (1986). 'Hospital routines in infants with hyper-bilirubinaemia influence the duration of breastfeeding'. *Acta Paediatr. Scand.* 75: p.708

Enzunga, A., Fischer, P.R. (1990). 'Neonatal weight loss in rural Zaire'. *Ann Trop Paediatr.* 10.

Fildes, op. cit. pp.48 - 52, pp.168-83 .

Fildes, V. (1986). *Breasts, Bottles and Babies: A History of Infant Feeding.* Edinburgh: Edinburgh University Press. pp.118 -120, 139-44.

Filteau, S.M., Tompkins, A.M. (1995). 'Vitamin A supplementation in developing countries'. *Arch Dis Child,* 72: pp.106-07.

Fisher, C. (1993). 'Feeding'. In: Bennet, V.R., Brown, I.K. (Eds.) *Myles Textbook for Midwives.* Edinburgh: Churchill Livingstone. 12th edn. p.523.

Fisher, M.C. (1992). 'Blocked ducts'. *New Generation.* 1(1):16-17.

Food Chemical News (1985). June 17th.

Forsyth, S. (1992). 'More evidence of the benefits is required'. *Pulse of Medicine,* June 6:57-8.

Fransson, G.B. (1980). 'Iron in human milk'. *J. Pediatr.* 96: pp.380-84.

Freeborn, S.F., Calvert, R.T., Black, P. et al. (1980). 'Saliva and blood pethidine concentrations in the mother and newborn baby'. *British Journal of Obstetrics and Gynacology.* 87: pp.966-69.

Garforth, S., Garcia, J. (1989). 'Breastfeeding policies in practice - No wonder they get confused'. *Midwifery,* 5: pp.75-83.

Gartner, L.M., Arias, I.M. (1987). 'Temporary discontinuation of breastfeeding in infants with jaundice'. *JAMA;* 225: p.532.

Gartner, L.M., Lee, K.S. (1980). 'Effect of starvation and milk feeding on intestinal bilirubin absorption'. *Pediatr. Res.* 14: p.498.

Garza, C., Johnson, C.A., Harrist, R. et. al. (1982). 'Effects of methods of collection and storage on nutrients in human milk.' *Early Human Dev.* 6: pp.295-303.

Ghana, VAST Study Team (1993). 'Vitamin A supplementation in northern Ghana: effects on clinic attendances, hospital admission and child mortality'. *Lancet,* 342: pp.7-12.

Gittleman, I.F., Pincus, J.B. (1951). 'Influence of diet on occurrence of hyperphosphatemia and hypocalcaemia in the newborn infant'. *Pediatrics;* 8: pp.778-86.

Glasier, A., McNeilly, A.S., Howie, P.W. (1984). 'The prolactin response to suckling'. *Clinical Endocrinology,* 12: pp.109-16.

Glass, R.I. et. al. (1983). 'Protection against Cholera in breastfed children by antibodies in breastmilk'. *New Engl. J. Med.* 308; pp.1289-92.

Goldblum, R.M., Garza, C., Johnson, C. et. al. (1981). 'Human milk banking 1: Effects of container upon immunologic factors in mature milk'. *Nutr. Res.* 1: pp.449-59.

Golding, J., Greenwood, R., Birmingham, K., Mott, L. (1992). 'Childhood cancer, Vitamin K and pethidine given during labour'. *BMJ:* 305: pp.341-46.

Goldman, A.S., Atkinson, S.A., Hanson, L.A. (1987). *Human Lactation,* Vol. 3, New York: Plenum.

Goldman, A.S., Goldblum, R.M. (1989). 'Immunologic systems in Human milk: characteristics and effects'. In: Lebenthal, E. (Ed.) *Textbook of Gastro-enterology and Nutrition in Early Pregnancy.* 2nd Edn. pp.135-42, New York: Raven Press.

Gottleib, E. (1992). 'Blocked ducts'. *New Generation.* 1(1): 16-17.

Graffy, J. (1992). 'Mothers' attitudes to and experience of breastfeeding: a primary care study'. *British Journal of General Practice* 42: pp.61-64.

Greenberg, F.K. et al. (1973). 'First mothers rooming-in with their newborns: its impact on mothers'. *Am J Orthopsychiatry,* 43: pp.783-88.

Gunther, M. (1945). 'Sore nipples: causes and prevention', *Lancet,* 2: pp.590-93.

Hall, M. (1984). 'Antenatal care: Are our accepted practices based on valid assumptions?' In: Zander, L., Chamberlain, G. (Eds.) *Pregnancy Care for the 1980s.* London: RSM and Macmillan Press. p.3.

Hambraeus, L. (1977). 'Proprietary milk versus human breast milk in infant feeding'. *Paediatric Clin North Am;* 24: pp.17-36.

Hambraeus, L., Forsum, E., Loennerdal, B. (1976). 'Nutritional aspects of breastmilk versus cows' milk formulas'. In: MacFarlane, H., Hambraeus, L., Hanson, L.A. (Eds.). *Food and Immunology.* Symposia of the Swedish Nutrition Foundation XIII. Stockholm, Sweden: Almqvist and Wiksell.

Hansen, T.W.R., Bratlid, D. (1986). 'Bilirubin and brain toxicity'. *Acta Paediatr. Scand.* 75; p.513.

Harzer, G., Dieterich, I., Haug, M. (1984). 'Effects of the diet on composition of human milk'. *Ann.Nutr. Metab.* 28: p.231.

Hawdon, J., Ward Platt, M.P., Aynsley-Green, A. (1993). 'Neonatal hypo-glycaemia - blood glucose monitoring and baby feeding'. *Midwifery*, 9; p.3-6.

Hawdon, J.M., Ward Platt, M.P., Aynsley-Green, A. (1992). 'Patterns of metabolic adaptation in term and preterm infants in the first postnatal week'. *Arch. Dis. Child.* 67: pp.357-65.

Heaton, K.W. (1987). 'Aetiology of acute appendicitis'. *BMJ*, 294: pp.1632-33.

Heck, I.J., Erenberg. (1987). 'Serum glucose levels in term neonates during the first 48 hours of life'. *J Pediatr*, 110: pp.119-22.

Hewat, R.J., Ellis, D.J. (1987). 'A comparison of the effectiveness of two methods of nipple care'. *Birth*: 14 (1), pp.41-45.

Hewitt, M. (1958). *Wives and Mothers in Victorian Industry*, London: pp.137-38.

Hey, E. (1995). 'Neonatal jaundice - how much do we really know?' *Midwifery Digest*, Vol. 5, No.1, March, pp.4-8.

Hill, A.F. (1968). 'A salute to La Leche League International'. *J. Pediatr*, 73, pp.161-2.

Holmes, T.H., Rahe, R.H. (1967). 'Social readjustment rating scale'. *Journal Psychosomatic Res.*; 11: p.219.

Host, A. (1991). 'Importance of the first meal on the develoment of cow's milk allergy and intolerance'. *Allergy Proc*; 12: pp.227-32.

Host, A., Husby, S., Osterballe, O.A. (1988). 'Prospective study of cows' milk allergy in exclusively breastfed infants'. *Acta paediatr Scand*; 77: pp.663-70.

Houston, M.J. et al. (1983). 'Factors affecting the duration of breastfeeding: Measurement of breastmilk intake in the first week of life'. *Early Hum Dev*; 8: pp.49-54.

Howie, P.W. et. al. (1982). 'Fertility after childbirth: infant feeding patterns, basal prolactin levels and postpartum ovulation'. *Clin. Endocrinol.* 17: pp.315-22.

Howie, P.W., Forsyth, J.S., Ogston, S.A., Clark, A., Florey C du V. (1990). 'Protective effect of breastfeeding against infection', *BMJ*; 300: pp.11-16.

Howie, P.W., McNeilly, A.S. (1980). 'The initiation of lactation'. *Midwife, Health Visitor and Community Nurse.* April, pp.142-44.

Howie, P.W., McNeilly, A.S., McArdle, T., Smart, L., Houston, M. (1980b). 'The relation between suckling-induced prolactin response and lactogenesis'. *J. Clin. Endocrinol. Metab.* 50; pp.670-73.

Hoyle, D. (1992). 'Blocked ducts'. *New Generation.* 1(1): 16-17.

Hunter, M. (1994). 'Counselling in obstetrics and gynaecology'. *The British Psychological Society*, 104;

Illingworth, R., Illingworth, A. (1956). *Babies and Young Children. Feeding: Management: Care.* J. and A. Churchill Ltd: pp.45, 48, 65.

Illingworth, R.S., Stone, D.G. (1952). 'Self-demand feeding in a maternity unit'. *Lancet i:* pp.683-87.

Inch, S. (1990). 'Postnatal care relation to breastfeeding'. In: Alexander, J., Levy, V., Roch, S. (Eds.) *Midwifery Practice: Postnatal Care.* Macmillan Education Ltd. p.33.

Inch, S., Fisher, C. (1993). 'The Avent Niplette - is it of value?' *AIMS Journal*; 5 (4): pp.13-14.

Inch, S., Garforth, S. (1998). 'Establishing and maintaining breastfeeding'. In: Chalmers, I., Enkin, M. W., Kierse, M. (Eds.) *Effective Care in Pregnancy and Childbirth.* Oxford: Oxford University Press. pp.1359-74.

Inch, S., Renfrew, M.J. (1989). 'Common breastfeeding problems'. In: Chalmers, I., Enkin, M., Kierse, M. (Eds). *Effective Care in Pregnancy and Childbirth*. Oxford: Oxford University Press. p.1375.

Jain, N., Mathur, N.B., Sharma, V.K., Dwarkadas, A.M. (1991). 'Cellular composition including lymphocyte subsets in preterm and full term human colostrum and milk', *Acta Paediatr Scand* 80: pp.395-99.

Jakobsson, I., Lindberg, T. (1983). 'Cows' milk proteins cause infantile colic in breastfed infants; a double blind cross-over study'. *Pediatrics*, 71(2); pp.268-71.

Jelliffe, P., Jelliffe, E.F.P. (1988). *Programmes to Promote Breastfeeding*. Oxford Medical Publications, Oxford University Press. p.4.

Jensen, R., Jensen, G. (1992). 'Specialty Lipids for infant nutrition. 1. milks and formulas' *J. Pediatr. Gastroenterol Nutr.* 15: pp.232-45.

Jesuru, C.A., Ostrea, E.M. (1979). 'Elevated serum bilirubin and albumin saturation in breastfed infants: role of supplemental feedings'. *Pediatr Res*; 13: p.497A.

Karjaleinen, J., Martin, J.M., Knip, M., Ilonen, J., Robinson, B.H., Savilahti, E., Akerblom, H.K., Dosch, H-M. (1992). 'A bovine albumin peptide as a possible trigger of insulin-dependent diabetes mellitus'. *New Engl J Med*. 327: pp.302-07.

Keefe, R.M. (1987). 'Comparison of neonatal night time sleep-wake patterns in nursery versus rooming-in environments'. *Nursing Research*; 36: pp.140-44.

Kemper, K., Forsyth, B., McCarthy, P. (1989). 'Jaundice, terminating breast-feeding and the vulnerable child'. *Pediatrics*, 84: pp.773-77.

Kendall, S. (1995). *Invest in Breast Together*. Health Visitors Association and Royal College of Midwives.

Kennedy, K.I. et. al. (1989). 'Consensus statement on the use of breastfeeding as a family planning method'. *Contraception*; 39: p.477.

Kennedy, P. (1982). 'Blocked ducts - revisited'. *New Generation*. 1(4): 16-19.

Kirkpatrick, C.T. (1992). *Illustrated Handbook of Medical Physiology*. Chichester.:John Wiley & Sons. p.535.

Klaus, Farnaroff. (1979. 'Care of the high-risk neonate', Philadelphia: W.B. Saunders Co.

Klaus, M.H., Jerauls, R., Kreger, N., McAlpine, W., Steffa, M., Kennel, J.H. (1972). 'Maternal attachment: importance of the first post-partum days'. *New England Journal of Medicine*; 284: pp.460-3.

Klaus, M.H., Kennell, J.H. (1982). *Parent-Infant Bonding*. The C.V. Mosby Company: pp.40, 48-49.

Kleigman, R.M. (1979). 'Neonatal necrotising enterocolitis: implications for an infectious disease'. *Pediatr Clin North Am*; 26: pp.327-44.

Koh, T.H.H.G., Eyre, J.A., Aynsley Green, A. (1988). 'Neonatal hypoglycaemia - the controversy regarding definition'. *Arch Dis Child*; 63: pp.1386-88.

Koppe, J.G. et al. (1989). 'Breastmilk, PCBs, dioxins and vitamin K deficiency: discussion paper'. *Journal of the Royal Society of Medicine*; 82: pp.416-19.

Kries, V.R, Shearer, M., McCarthy, P.T., Haug, M., Harzer, G., Goebel, U. (1987). 'Vitamin K Content of Maternal Milk: Influence of the Stage of Lactation, Lipid Composition, and Vitamin K Supplements Given to the Mother'. *Paediatric Research*; 22, 5: pp.513-17.

Kroeger, M. (1993). *Labor and Delivery Practices: The 11th Step to Successful Breastfeeding*, International Confederation of Midwives 23rd Congress, Vancouver.

Kron, R.E., Stein, M., Goddard, K.E. (1966). 'Newborn sucking behaviour affected by obstetric medication'. *Pediatrics;* 87: pp.1012-16.

Kuhr, M., Paneth, N. (1982). 'Feeding practices and early neonatal jaundice'. *J Pediatr Gastroenterol Nutr.* 1: pp.485-88.

Lane, P., Hathaway, W.E. (1985). 'Vitamin K in infancy'. *J. Pediatr,* 106: pp.351-60.

Lanting, C.I. et.al. (1994). 'Neurological differences between 9-year-old children fed breastmilk and formula milk as babies'. *The Lancet,* 344: pp.1319-22.

Larson, E., Zuill, R., Zier, V. et. al. (1984). 'Storage of human breast milk'. *Infection Control* 5: pp.127-30.

Lawrence, R. (1989). *Breastfeeding, A Guide for the Medical Profession.* 4th Edn. New York: CV Mosby. p.66.

Lawrence, R. A. (1994). *Breastfeeding: A Guide for the Medical Profession.* The C.V. Mosby Company: p.392.

Lawrence, R.A. (1989). *Breastfeeding - A Guide For The Medical Profession,* 3rd Ed. pp.126-127. C.V. Mosby Company.

Lawrence, R.A. (1994). *Breastfeeding - A Guide For The Medical Profession,* 4th Ed. pp. 1, 42, 104, 113, 203-4, 285, 452-3. C.V. Mosby Company.

Lawson, M. (1992). 'Non-nutritional factors in human breastmilk'. *Modern Midwife,* Nov/Dec: pp.18-21.

Leake, R.D., Waters, C.B., Rubin, R.T. et. al. (1983). 'Oxytocin and prolactin responses in long-term breastfeeding'. *Obstetric Gynecol* 62; p.565.

Liebig, J. (1843). *Animal Chemistry.* 2nd ed., translated into English by W. Gregory, London: Taylor and Walton.

Lindenberg, C et al. (1990). 'The effect of early post-partum mother-infant contact and breastfeeding promotion on the incidence and continuation of breastfeeding', *Int J Nurs Stud;* 27: pp.179-86.

Linzell, J.L., Peaker, M. (1971). 'Mechanism of milk secretion'. *Physiological Reviews* 51: pp.564-97.

Lodge, J. (1982). 'Blocked ducts - revisited'. *New Generation.* 1(4): 16-19.

Lucas, A. et. al. (1992). 'Breastmilk and subsequent intelligent quotient in children born preterm'. *Lancet,* 339: pp.261-64.

Lucas, A. et.al. (1991). letter. *Br. Med. J.* 302:351 -1

Lucas, A. et.al. (1992). 'Randomized trial of a ready-to-feed compared with powdered formula'. *Arch. Dis. Child.* 67: pp.935-39.

Lucas, A., Cole, T.J. (1990). 'Breast milk and neonatal necrotising enterocolitis.' *The Lancet;* 336: pp.1519-23.

Macaulay, D., Watson, M. (1967). 'Hypernatraemia in infants as a cause of brain damage'. *Arch Dis Child;* 42: pp.485-91.

MAFF (1981). *The Food Standard Committee Report on Infant Formulae (Artificial feeds for the young infant).* FSC/REP/73. London: HMSO.

Maisels, M.J., Gifford, K. (1983). 'Breastfeeding weight-loss and jaundice'. *J Pediatr,* 102: pp.117-18.

Maisels, M.J., Gifford, K. (1986). 'Normal serum bilirubin levels in the newborn and the effect on breastfeeding'. *Pediatrics,* 78 (5): pp.837-43.

Maisels, M.J., Gifford, K., Antle, C.B., Leib, G.R. (1985). 'Jaundice in the healthy newborn infant: a new approach to an old problem'; *Pediatrics,* 81: pp.505-11.

Maisels, M.J., Vain, N., Acquavita, A.M,, de Blanco, N.V., Cohen, A., DiGregorio, J. (1991). 'The effect of breastfeeding frequency on serum bilirubin levels'. *Am. J. Obstet. Gynecol:* 170; pp.880-83.

Makrides, M. et.al. (1994). 'Fatty acid composition of brain, retina, and erythrocytes in breast and formula-fed infants'. 60: p.189.

Martin, J. (1978). *Infant Feeding 1975. Survey carried out for the DHSS by the Office of Population Censuses and Surveys.* London: HMSO.

Martin, J., Monk, J. (1982). *Infant Feeding 1980; Office of Population Censuses and Surveys.* London: HMSO.

Martin, J., White, A. (1988). *Infant Feeding 1985. Office of Population Censuses and Surveys.* London: HMSO.

Martinez, J. et al. (1993). 'Hyperbilirubinaemia in the breastfed newborn: a controlled trial of four interventions'. *Pediatrics* 91: pp.470-73.

Matthews, M. K. (1989). 'The relationship between maternal labour analgesia and delay in the initiation of breastfeeding in healthy neonates in the early neonatal period'. *Midwifery*, 5: pp.3-10.

McCance, R.A., Widdowson, E.M. (1957). 'Hypertonic expansion of the extracellular fluid'. *Acta Paed*, 46: pp.337-53.

McCandish, R., Renfrew, M., Alexander, J. (1993). Letter; *Midwives Chronicle and Nursing Notes*; November, p.1433.

McGeorge, D.M. (1993). The 'Niplette. An instrument for the non-surgical correction of inverted nipples'. *Brit J of Plastic Surgery*, 47, pp.46-49.

McNeilly, A.S. et.al. (1983). 'Fertility after childbirth: pregnancy associated with breastfeeding'. *Clin Endocrinol*,18: p.167.

Messenger, H. (1994). 'Don't shoot the messenger'. *Health visitor*, 67 (5) May p.171.

Minchin, M. (1985). *Breastfeeding Matters.* Australia: Alma Publications and George Allen and Unwin. pp.11, 150.

Minchin, M. (1987). 'Infant formula: A mass, uncontrolled trial in perinatal care'. *Birth*; 14: pp.25-33.

Ministry of Health (1943). *Report on The Breast Feeding of Infants.* London: HMSO. p. 2, p. 9. (Reports on public health and medical subjects; No 91).

Ministry of Health (1944). *The Breastfeeding Infants - Report of the Advisory Committee on Mothers and Children.* London: HMSO, pp.13.

Miranda, R., Saravia, N.G., Ackerman, R. et. al. (1983). 'Effect of maternal nutritional status on immunological substances in colostrum and milk'. *Am. J. Clin. Nutr.* 37; p.632.

Montagu, A. (1986). *Touching - The Human Significance of Skin.* 3rd Edition. Perennial Library. New York: Harper and Row, pp.70-71.

Morrow-Tlucak M. et. al. (1988). 'Breastfeeding and cognitive development in the first two years of life'. *Soc Sci Med* 26: pp.635-39.

Murray, A.D. et al. (1981). 'Effects of epidural anaesthesia on newborns and their mothers'. *Child Development*, 52: pp.71-82

Myles, M. F. (1961). *A Textbook for Midwives.* E. and S. Livingstone Ltd, p.522.

Myles, M.F. (1985). *Textbook for Midwives.* 10th Ed. Edinburgh: Churchill Livingstone. p.540.

National Academy of Sciences (1991). *Nutrition During Lactation.* Washington DC: National Academy Press. p.121.

Neibyl, J.R., Spence, M.R., Parmley, T.H. (1978). 'Sporadic (non-epidemic) puerperal mastitis'. *Journal of Reproductive Medicine*; 20: pp.97-100.

Neifert, M.R., Seacat, J.M., Jobe, W.E. (1986). 'Lactation failure due to insufficient glandular development of the breast.' *Paediatrics*, 76; pp.823-28.

Nemethy, M., Clore, E.R. (1990). 'Microwave heating of infant formula and breastmilk.' *Journal Pediatr Hlth Care.* 4: pp.131-35.

Newcomb, P.A. et.al. (1994). 'Lactation and a reduced risk of pre-menopausal breast cancer'. *New England J Med,* 33: pp.81-87.

Newman, T.B., Maisels, M.J. (1992). 'Evaluation and treatment of jaundice in the term newborn: a kinder gentler approach'. *Pediatrics,* 80: p.809.

Newton, M., Newton, N.R. (1948). 'The Let-down reflex in human lactation'. *J. Pediatrics,* 33 (6); pp.698-704.

Newton, N. (1952). 'Nipple pain and nipple damage'. *Journal of Paediatrics,* 41: pp.411-23.

Nicodem, V.C., Danziger, D., Gebka, N., Gulmezoglu, A.M., Hofmeyr, G.J. (1994). 'Do cabbage leaves prevent engorgement? A RCT Study'. *Birth,* 20; pp.61-64

Nicoll, A., Ginsburg, R., Tripp, J.H. (1982). 'Supplementary feeding and jaundice in newborns'. *Acta Pediatr Scand.* 71: pp.759-61.

Nwankwo, M.U., Offor, E., Okolo, A.A. et. al (1988). 'Bacterial growth in expressed breastmilk'. *Ann Trop Peadiatr.* 8: pp.92-95.

Odent, M. (1984). *Birth Reborn.* New York: Pantheon Books, p.73.

Oppe, T.E., Redstone, D. (1968). 'Calcium and phosphorus levels in healthy newborn infants given various types of milk'. *Lancet* i: pp.1045-48.

Osborn, L.M., Lenarsky, C., Oakes, R.C. et. al. (1984). 'Phototherapy in fullterm infants with haemolytic disease secondary to ABO incompatibility'. *Pediatrics,* 74: pp.371-74.

Oski, F.A. (1985). 'Is bovine milk a health hazard?' *Pediatrics* 75; (part 2): pp.182-86.

Oski, F.A. (1988). 'Physiological jaundice'. In: Avery, M.E., Taeusch, H.W. Jnr, (Eds.) *Diseases of the Newborn.* 5th Edn. Philadelphia: PA. WB Saunders.

Palmer, G. (1993). 'The Mabel Liddiard Lecture, 'Who helps health professionals with breastfeeding?' *Midwives Chronicle.* May. pp.147-56.

Parker, C. (1994). 'Research and quality assurance issues'; *British Journal of Midwifery* 2: p.60.

Peaker, M., Wilde, C.J. (1987). 'Milk secretion: autocrine control'. *News Physiol. Sci.* 2: p.12406.

Perez, A. et al. (1992). 'Clinical study of the lactational amenorrhoea method of family planning'. *The Lancet,* 339: p.968.

Piscane, et.al. (1995). 'Breastfeeding and acute appendicitis'. *BMJ,* 310: pp.836-7.

Pitt, B. (1978). *Feelings about Childbirth,* London: Sheldon Press.

Pittard, W.B., Anderson, D.M., Cerutti, E.R. et. al. (1985). 'Bacteriostatic qualities of human milk.' *J. Pediatr.* 107: pp.240-43.

Prentice, A.M. et al. (1984). 'Breastmilk antimicrobial factors of rural Gambian mothers'. *Acta Paediatr.* Scand. 73; pp.796 - 812.

Prentice, A.M., Addey, C.V.P., Wilde, C.J. (1989). 'Evidence for local feed-back control of human milk secretion'. *Biochemical Society Transactions* 17, p.122, 489-92.

Prentice, A.M., Prentice, A. (1988). 'Energy cost of lactation.' *Annu Rev Nutr,* 8: p.63.

Present Day Practice in Infant feeding (1974). *DHSS Report on Health and Social Subjects* 9, HMSO: London.

Procianoy, R.S. et al. (1983). 'The influence of rooming-in on breastfeeding'. *Journal of Tropical Paediatrics* 29; pp.112-14.

Pugh, R.J. (1981). 'Allergy to cow's milk protein'. *Health Visitor,* 54: pp.231-33.

Purves, C. (1982). 'Blockeed ducts - revisited'. *New Generation.* 1(4): 16-19.

Quan, R.., Yang, C., Rubinstein, S. et. al. (1992). 'Effects of microwave radiation on anti-infective factors in human milk'. *Pediatr.* 89: pp.667-69.

Rahi, J.S et al. (1995). 'Childhood blindness due to vitamin A deficiency in India: regional variations'. *Arch Dis Child.* 72: pp.330-33.

Rajan, L. (1993). 'Perceptions of pain and pain relief in labour: the gulf between experience and observation', *Midwifery*, 9, pp.136-45.

Rajan, L. (1993). 'The contribution of professional support, information and consistent advice to successful breastfeeding'. *Midwifery*, 9: pp.197-209.

Rajan, L. (1994). 'The impact of obstetric procedures and analgesia/anaesthesia during labour and delivery on breastfeeding'. *Midwifery*, 10: pp.87-103.

RCM (1991). *Successful Breastfeeding - a Handbook for Midwives.* 2nd Edn. Edinburgh: Churchill Livingstone, p.53.

Read, G.D. (1954). *Childbirth Without Fear.* London: William Heineman. pp. 161-62.

Renfrew, M.J., Fisher, M.C., Arms, S. (1990). *Bestfeeding - Getting Breastfeeding Right for You.* Berkeley: Celestial Arts. pp.89-94.

Righard, L., Alade, M.O. (1992). 'Sucking technique and its effect on success of breastfeeding'. *Birth* 19: 4 December: pp.187-89.

Righard, L., Alade, O. M. (1990). 'Effects of delivery room routines on success of first feed'. *The Lancet*, 336: pp.1105-07.

Riordan, J., Auerbach, K. (1993). *Breastfeeding and Human Lactation.* Boston/London: Jones and Bartlett. p.82.

Robert, A. (1979). 'Cytoprotection by prostaglandins'. *Gastroenterology,* 77: pp.761-67.

Robert, Woodward, J. (1984). *Urban Disease and Mortality in 19th Century England,* London: Batsford.

Robertson, K.J. (1993). 'Neonatal jaundice - mechanism and diagnosis'. *Modern Midwife*, 3(5): pp.28-33.

Rosier, W. (1988). 'Cool cabbage compresses' *Breastfeeding Review*, 12; p.28.

Royal College of Midwives (1991). *Successful Breastfeeding.* Edinburgh: Churchill Livingstone; 2nd Edn., pp. 9-11, 62.

Saarinnen, U.M., Slimes, M.A. (1979). 'Iron absorption from breast milk, cow's milk and iron supplemented formula: an opportunistic use of changes in total body iron determined by haemoglobin, ferritin and body weight in 132 infants', *Pediatr. res.* 13: pp.143-47.

Saint, L., Maggiore, P., Hartmann, P.E. (1986). 'Yield and nutrient content of milk in eight women breastfeeding twins and one woman breastfeeding triplets'. *British Journal of Nutrition* 56, pp.49-58.

Saint, L., Smith, M., Hartmann, P.E. (1984). 'The yield and content of colostrum and milk of women from giving birth to one month post-partum'. *British Journal of Nutrition.* 52; pp.87-95.

Salariya, E.M., Robertson, C.M. (1993). 'Relationships between baby feeding types and patterns, gut transit time of meconium and the incidence of neonatal jaundice'. *Midwifery*, 9: pp.235-42.

Salariya, E.M., Robertson, C.M. (1993b). 'The development of a neonatal stool colour comparator'. *Midwifery*, 9: pp.35-40.

Salaryia, E.M., Easton, P.M., Cater, J.I. (1978). 'Duration of feeding after early initiation and frequent feeding'. *Lancet ii*: pp.1141-43.

Schaffer, S.G. (1977). *Mothering.* London: Fontana Open Books. p. 39.

Schaffer, S.G. et al. (1987). 'Postnatal weight changes in low-birth-weight infants'. *Pediatrics*; 79: pp.702-05.

Schneider, A.P. (1986). 'Breastmilk and jaundice in the newborn - a real entity'. *JAMA*: 225: pp.3270-74.

Scowen, P. (1989). '1964 -1974; Bottle-feeding and early weaning reach a peak'. *Midwife, Health Visitor & Community Nurse;* 25: pp.293-305.

Secretary of State for Health (1992). *The Health of the Nation. A Strategy for Health in England.* London: HMSO.

Sharp, D. A. (1992). 'Moist wound healing for sore and cracked nipples'. *Breastfeeding Abstracts*; 12: p.19.

Shukla, A., Forsyth, H.A., Anderson, C.M., Marwah, S.M. (1972). 'Infantile over nutrition in the first year of life: a field study in Dudley, Worcestershire'. *BMJ*; iv: pp.12-15.

Sigman, M., Burke, K.I., Swarner, O.W. et. al. (1989). 'Effects of microwaving human milk: changes in IgA content and bacterial count'. *J. Amer. Diet. Assoc.* 89: pp.690-92.

Sinclair, A.J., Crawford, M.A. (1972). 'The accumulation of arachidonate and doxosahexaenate in the developing rat brain', *J Neurochem* 19: p.1753.

Sinclair, C.M. (1992). *Fats in Human milk. Topics in Breastfeeding* Set IV April 1992. Lactation Resource Centre.

Sloper, K., Elsden, E., Baum, J.D. (1977). 'Increasing breastfeeding in a community'. *Arch. Dis. Child.* 52: pp.700-02.

Snell, R.S. (1995). *Clinical Anatomy*, 5th Edition. London: Little, Brown & Co.

Sosa, R., Kennell, J.H., Klaus, M.H., Urrutia, J.J. (1976). 'The effect of early mother infant contact on breastfeeding, infection and growth'. In: *Breastfeeding and The Mother.* Elsevier, Amsterdam: Ciba foundation Symposium 45.

Spence, J.C. (1938). 'The modern decline of breast-feeding'. *Br Med J*; 2: pp.729-33.

Spock , B. (1969). *Baby and Child Care.* The Bodley Head. pp.68-69.

Standing Committee on Nutrition of the British Paediatric Association (1994). 'Is breastfeeding beneficial in the UK?' *Archives of Diseases of Childhood,* 71: pp.376 -80.

Stanway, A. P. (1982). *The Breast. A Mayflower Book.* London: Granada pp.35-37.

Stanway, A., Stanway, P. (1983). *Breast is Best.* London: Pan Books. 2nd Edn. pp. 55, 155, 244.

Stapleton, T. et al. (1957). 'The pathogenesis of idiopathic hypercalcaemia in infancy'. *Am. J. Clin. Nutr.* 5: pp.533-42.

Stechler, G. (1964). 'Newborn attention as affected by medication during labour'. *Science*; 144: pp.315-17.

Sweet, B. (1988). *A Textbook for Midwives.* 11th ed. London: Bailliere Tindall.

Taitz, L.S., Byers, H.D. (1972). 'High calorie/osmolar feeding and hypertonic dehydration'. *Arch Dis Child*; 47: pp.257-60.

Tarn, A.C., Thomas, J.M. (1988). 'Predicting insulin-dependent diabetes', *Lancet,* 1: pp.845-50.

Taylor, P. (1982). 'Blocked ducts - revisited'. *New Generation.* 1(4): 16-19.

Thomsen, A. C., Espersen, T., Maigaard, S. (1984). 'Course and treatment of milk stasis, non-infectious inflammation of the breast and infective mastitis in nursing women'. *Am. J. Obstet. Gynecol*; 149; pp.492-95.

Toole, G., Toole, S. (1993). 'Understanding biology - for advanced level', Cheltenham: Stanley Thornes Ltd. p.574.

Toothill, B. (1995). 'Infant feeding in a refugee camp'. *Midwives*, May, pp.150-151.

UNICEF (1990). *Innocenti Declaration*. UNICEF, Nutrition Cluster (H-8F), 3 United Nations Plaza, New York, N.Y.10017.USA.

United Kingdom National Case-Control Study Group (1993). 'Breast feeding and risk of breast cancer in young women'. *BMJ*, 307: pp.17-20.

Uuay, R.D. et. al. (1990). 'Effect of dietary Omega 3 fatty acids on retinal function of very low birthweight neonates'. *Pediatr. Res.* 28: pp.485-92.

Victora, C.G. et al. (1987). 'Evidence for protection by breast-feeding against infant deaths from infectious diseases in Brazil', *Lancet*, 2: pp.319-22.

Waldenstrom, U., Swenson, A. (1991). 'Rooming-in at night in the postpartum ward'; *Midwifery*, 7: pp.82-89.

West, C.P. (1980). 'Factors influencing the duration of breastfeeding'. *Journal Biosoc Sci.* 12: pp.325-31.

White, A., Freeth, S., O,Brien, M. (1992). *Infant feeding 1990. Survey carried out for the DHSS by the Office of Population Censuses and Surveys*. London: HMSO.

Whitehead, R.G., Paul, A.A. (1981). 'Infant growth and human milk requirements: a fresh approach'. *Lancet* 2: pp.161-63.

Whitehead, R.G., Paul, A.A. (1984). 'Growth charts and the assessment of infant feeding practices in the western world and in developing countries'. *Early Human Development*, 9; pp.187-207.

Whitfield, M.F., Kay, R., Stevens, S. (1981). 'Validity of routine clinical test weighing as a measure of the intake of breastfed infants'. *Archives of Disease of Childhood*, 56: pp.919-21.

WHO/UNICEF (1993). *Breastfeeding Counselling: A Training course. Trainer's Guide. Division of diarrhoeal and acute respiratory disease control;* Geneva. p.187.

Wilde, C.J., Addey, C.V.P., Casey, M.J., Blatchford, D.R., Peaker, M. (1988). 'Feed-back inhibition of milk secretion: the effect of a fraction of goat milk on milk yield and composition'. *Quarterly Journal of Experimental Physiology*, 73, pp.391-97.

Williams, A.F. (1994). 'Is breastfeeding beneficial in the UK? Statement of the Standing Committee on Nutrition of the British Paediatric Association.' *Arch Dis Child*, 71: pp.376-79.

Willmott, M.P., Colhoun, E.M., Bolton, A.E. (1977). 'The suppression of puerperal lactation with brompcriptine'. *Acta Obstet Gynecol Scand* 56: p.145.

Wolff, P.H. (1966). *The Causes, Controls,and Organization of Behaviour in the Neonate*. New York: International Universities Press.

Wood, B., Culley, P., Roginski, C. et. al. (1979). 'Factors affecting neonatal jaundice'. *Arch dis. child.* 54: pp.111-15.

Wood, C.B.S., Walker-Smith, J.A. (1981). *MacKeith's Infant Feeding and Feeding Difficulties*. 6th Edition. Edinburgh: Churchill Livingstone. p.3.

Woolridge, M. W. (1986). 'Aetiology of sore nipples'. *Midwifery*, 2: pp.172-76.

Woolridge, M. W. (1986b). 'The 'anatomy' of infant sucking'. *Midwifery*, 2: pp.164-71.

Woolridge, M.W. (1993). 'Clinical management of breastfeeding problems: The contented, failure-to-thrive breastfed baby revisited'. Abstract of a paper presented at the Annual conference of the Society for Reproductive and Infant Psychology. September, ISSN 0264 6838.

Woolridge, M.W., Baum, J.D. (1983). 'Recent advances in breastfeeding'. *Acta Paediatrica Japonica*, 35: pp.1-12.

Woolridge, M.W., Baum, J.D., Drewett, R.F. (1982). 'Individual patterns of milk intake during breastfeeding'. *Early Human Development*, 7: pp.265-72.

Woolridge, M.W., Fisher, M.C. (1988). 'Colic "overfeeding" and symptoms of lactose Malabsorption in the breastfed baby; a possible artifact of feed management?' *Lancet ii*, pp.382-84.

World Health Organization (1989). *Protecting, Promoting and Supporting Breast-Feeding: the Special Role of Maternity Services*. WHO, Geneva.

World Health Organization (1992). *Global Hospital Assessment (Questionnaire) for the WHO/UNICEF BFHI*. WHO: Geneva.

World Health Organization (1992). *Guide for Scoring the Global Hospital Assessment for the WHO/UNICEF BFHI*. WHO: Geneva.

World Health Organization (1992). *Hospital Self-Appraisal Tool for the WHO/UNICEF BFHI*. WHO: Geneva.

Worthington-Roberts, B., Williams, S.R. (1989). *Nutrition in Pregnancy and Lactation*. 4th Edn. USA:Times Mirror/Mosby. pp.98, 276.

Worthington-Roberts, B., Williams, S.R. (1993). *Nutrition in Pregnancy and Lactation*. p.318.

Yamauchi, Y.Y., Yamanouchi, I. (1990). 'Breast-feeding frequency during the first 24 hours after birth in full-term neonates'. *Pediatrics*, 86 (2); pp.171-75.

APPENDIX ONE

Summary of the International Code of Marketing of Breastmilk Substitutes

The code includes the following ten provisions:

1.   No advertising of these products to the public.

2.   No free samples to mothers.

3.   No promotion of products in health care facilities.

4.   No company mothercraft nurses to advise mothers.

5.   No gifts or personal samples to health workers.

6.   No words or pictures idealizing artificial feeding, including labels, should explain the benefits of breastfeeding and the costs and hazards associated with artificial feeding.

7.   Information to health workers should be scientific and factual.

8.   All information on artificial feeding, including labels should explain the benefits of breastfeeding and the costs and hazards associated with artificial feeding.

9.   Unsuitable products, such as sweetened condensed milk, should not be promoted for babies.

10.   All products should be of high quality and take account of the climatic and storage conditions of the country where they are used.

(World Health Organization, Geneva, 1981.)

Ten Steps to Successful Breastfeeding

A Joint WHO/UNICEF Statement

Every facility providing maternity services and care for newborn infants should:

1.   Have a written breastfeeding policy that is routinely communicated to all health care staff.

2.   Train all health care staff in skills necessary to implement this policy.

3.   Inform all pregnant women about the benefits and management of breastfeeding

4.   Help mothers initiate breastfeeding within half an hour of birth.

5.   Show mothers how to breastfeed, and how to maintain lactation even if they should be separated from their infants.

6.   Give newborn infants no food or drink other than breastmilk, unless medically indicated.

7.   Practise rooming-in – allow mothers and infants to remain together 24 hours a day.

8.   Encourage breastfeeding on demand.

9.   Give no artificial teats or pacifiers (also called dummies or soothers) to breastfeeding infants.

10. Foster the establishment of breastfeeding support groups and refer mothers to them on discharge from hospital or clinic.

APPENDIX THREE

Innocenti Declaration

The Innocenti Declaration on the Protection, Promotion and Support of Breastfeeding recognizes that breastfeeding is a unique process that:

- provides ideal nutrition for infants and contributes to their healthy growth and development

- reduces incidence and severity of infectious diseases, thereby lowering morbidity and mortality

- contributes to women's health by reducing the risk of breast and ovarian cancer, and by increasing the spacing between pregnancies

- provides social and economic benefits to the family and the nation

- provides most women with the satisfaction when successfully carried out and that

- recent research has found that these benefits increase with increased exclusiveness of breastfeeding during the first six months of life, and thereafter with increased duration with complementary foods

- programme interventions can result in positive changes in breastfeeding behaviour

We therefore declare that:

> As a global goal for optimal maternal and child health and nutrition, all women should be enabled to practice exclusive breastfeeding and all infants should be fed on breastmilk from birth to four-six months of age. Thereafter, children should continue to be breastfed, while receiving appropriate and adequate complementary foods for up to two years of age or beyond. This child feeding ideal is to be achieved by creating an appropriate environment of awareness and support so that women can breastfeed in this manner.

This declaration was adopted by the participants at the WHO/UNICEF meeting *Breastfeeding in the 1990s: A Global Initiative*, co-sponsored by the United States Agency for International Development (USAID) and the Swedish International Development (SIDA) held at the Spedale degli Innocenti, Florence, Italy on 30 July - 1 August 1990.

Index